NEUROSCIENCE RESEARCH PROGRESS

MULTIPARAMETRIC IMAGING IN NEURODEGENERATIVE DISEASE

NEUROSCIENCE RESEARCH PROGRESS

Additional books and e-books in this series can be found on Nova's website under the Series tab.

NEUROSCIENCE RESEARCH PROGRESS

MULTIPARAMETRIC IMAGING IN NEURODEGENERATIVE DISEASE

YONGXIA ZHOU

nova
Medicine & Health
New York

Additional color graphics may be available in the e-book version of this book.

Library of Congress Cataloging-in-Publication Data

ISBN: 978-1-53615-338-5

Published by Nova Science Publishers, Inc. † New York

Contents

Preface		**vii**
Chapter 1	Introduction and Application of Neuroimaging Including Functional Neuronal Network in Neurodegenerative Disease	**1**
Chapter 2	Abnormal Functional Connectivity Network in Mild Traumatic Brain Injury, Post-Traumatic Stress Disorder, Mild Cognitive Impairment and Multiple Sclerosis	**23**
Chapter 3	Homotopic Imaging and Correlations with Neurocognitive Tests in Mild Traumatic Brain Injury, Post-Traumatic Stress Disorder, Mild Cognitive Impairment and Multiple Sclerosis	**65**
Chapter 4	Abnormal Microstructural Connectivity and Morphometry in Mild Traumatic Brain Injury, Post-Traumatic Stress Disorder, Mild Cognitive Impairment and Multiple Sclerosis	**107**

Chapter 5	Abnormal Molecular Imaging Including Tau, Amyloid and FDG in Mild Traumatic Brain Injury, Post-Traumatic Stress Disorder, Mild Cognitive Impairment and Multiple Sclerosis	**129**
Chapter 6	More Applications of Neuroimaging in Therapeutic Evaluation and New Horizon	**151**
Chapter 7	Summary of Multiparametric Imaging Results	**167**
About the Author		**175**
Index		**177**
Related Nova Publications		**191**

PREFACE

Post-traumatic stress disorder (PTSD) is a psychiatric disorder characterized by intrusions or re-experiencing, avoidance, hyperarousal and negative alterations in cognition and mood, commonly caused by traumatic exposure to warfare, traffic accident or abuse. Re-experiencing, avoidance and hyper-arousal are the typical symptoms of PTSD. Rates of comorbid PTSD and mild traumatic brain injury (MTBI) are estimated to be about 30% for TBI positive patients. Depending on type of exposure and gender, for instance, 16% of children who had been exposed to a traumatic event had developed PTSD. MTBI is a significant public health problem, representing 75% of the total TBI cases. The diagnosis inclusion criteria of MTBI include closed head injury with either posttraumatic amnesia of less than 24 hours or loss of consciousness of approximately 30 minutes or less, with a Glasgow Coma Scale score between 13 and 15. Thalamus as well as its frontal and temporal projections might be injured after TBI due to the relay central station function in brain. The commonly reported sequelae following trauma of any severity include fatigue, problems with sleep, problems with appetite and arousal, and lack of motivation, which are all closely related to hypothalamic dysfunction and neuropeptide dysregulation.

One of the hallmarks of Alzheimer's disease (AD) is amyloid pathology within the cerebral cortex accompanied by cortical thinning, structural reorganization, and recruitment of new areas for functional adaptation at early or preclinical stages of disease including mild cognitive impairment (MCI). The earliest neuropathologic changes including amyloid plaques and tau tangles associated with MCI/AD occur in the entorhinal and hippocampal cortices. Multiple sclerosis (MS) is a chronic inflammatory demyelinating disease that affects the whole brain. Neuroimaging techniques that can help elucidate and characterize the nature and mechanism of tissue injury and disease progression in MS are of particular importance given its roles in seeking successful preventive and therapeutic treatments of the disease. Imaging biomarkers of MS include multiple lesions, brain atrophy and normal appearing brain tissue abnormalities. There are quite a few recently developed advanced neuroimaging techniques including fMRI for detecting brain abnormalities such as default mode network (DMN) dysfunction, hippocampal, thalamic, hypothalamic injury and disruption of network connections, diffusion tensor imaging (DTI) for microstructure integrity analysis, and PET molecular tracers including tau, amyloid and FDG-glucose for underlying neuropathological burden quantification.

Multiple neuroimaging metrics will be demonstrated in this book to identify and quantify significant and distinct brain alterations at function, microstructure, morphology and molecular scales in different types of neurodegenerative diseases with high sensitivity and specificity. These comprehensive imaging features could be combined to improve disease diagnosis accuracy. The aim of this book is thus intended to provide both beginners and experts in biomedical imaging and health care a broad and complete picture as well as the new developments of using multiple metrics in improving disease identification, classification and therapeutic efficacy. This book would hopefully capture the interests of colleagues and researchers interested in the areas of neurodegenerative disease diagnosis and treatment, and could help convey the methodological and integrative perspectives of multiparametric neuroimaging applications.

Chapter 1 introduces the neurobiology and related imaging findings of the four representative neurodegenerative diseases, including brain region-specific disease related alterations, unique clinical symptom of each disease. There is an increasing body of literature which suggests that damage to the DMN, hypothalamus, thalamus and hippocampus functional connectivity based MRI (fcMRI) might been under-diagnosed and may account for some of the sequelae following the neurodegenerative injuries including PTSD, MTBI, MCI and MS. The purpose of Chapter 2 is to identify specific neuronal network abnormalities connecting from the four critical regions and any local activity injuries using advanced quantitative MRI techniques including the fcMRI. For instance, fcMRI results support the concept that functional networks of DMN, thalamic, hypothalamic and hippocampal connectivity, frontal and temporal cortical functional activity are altered after MTBI or PTSD at variable degrees. And in PTSD patients, various abnormal functional activity and connectivities had been observed, including decreased DMN and hippocampal fcMRI but increased hypothalamic and ventromedial prefrontal cortex (vmPFC) connectivity, with compensated cerebellar and occipital activations but lower activities in vmPFC, hippocampus and amygdala. Lower activity with higher functional connectivity suggested possible regional injuries and pathway compensation from surrounding areas or through structural connections.

Previous studies had shown good correspondence between homotopy imaging and myelin map. Chapter 3 had examined the functional homotopic differences in four neurodegenerative diseases including PTSD, MTBI, MCI and MS compared to controls; and further explore the correlations between quantitative voxel-mirrored homotopic correlation (VMHC) values and various neurocognitive/neuropsychological tests in patients. For instance, PTSD patients had lower homotopic connections in the parietal, temporal, thalamic radiation and optic radiation, with higher homotopic connections in vmPFC compared to controls ($P < 0.01$). Different VMHC pattern of MTBI was found with patients showing lower VMHC values in the hippocampus, bilateral dorsolateral prefrontal, temporal and occipital cortices but similarly higher VMHC in vmPFC. The brain regions that had lower homotopic values in PTSD patients were associated significantly with clinical symptoms.

In addition to identifying the functional network differences of the neurodegenerative diseases, Chapter 4 investigated the microstructural DTI imaging and other morphological brain changes including volumetry under disease conditions; and explored the graph-theory based small-worldness (SMW) differences in these patients compared to controls. Microstructural fractional anisotropy (FA) metric identified disease-specific alterations in patients, including uncinate, major forceps, corticospinal and cingulum tracts deterioration in PTSD; significant fornix and hippocampal cingulum FA reduction in MCI; diffuse axonal injury in the frontal and occipital cortices as well as corpus callosum in MTBI; and lower FA in the corpus callosum and optic radiation in MS patients. Similar characteristics in PTSD and AD/MCI patients, including local efficiency and small-worldness decreases but global efficiency increases were identified in contrast to the no SMW differences in MS patients, and higher local efficiency but lower global efficiency in MTBI patients compared to controls. Chapter 5 had quantified further available molecular imaging tracers such as tau, amyloid and FDG-glucose in the four neurodegenerative diseases. The results had shown significant differences of imaging biomarkers for detecting neurodegenerative diseases from controls. Distinct patterns of tau and amyloid depositions in MCI patients (e.g., higher tau at Braak stage II in MCI) compared to PTSD/TBI (higher tau at later Braak stages in PTSD, higher tau and amyloid in the vmPFC and temporal regions) were exhibited. And hypometabolism of glucose in PTSD and MCI had been found as well.

Then Chapter 6 reviewed some of the therapeutic effects of traditional Chinese medicine with neuroimaging quantifications to help treating neurodegenerative diseases and applying imaging techniques in other challenging diseases including cancer. Chapter 7 summarized the imaging findings and neural correlations with clinical data as well as treatment evaluations in previous chapters. Finally, an integrated neurobiology model of the pathological processes such as accumulation of tau, amyloid (Aβ), demyelination and dysfunction in specific regions and networks in these neurodegenerative diseases was proposed for better diagnosis and treatment.

Chapter 1 – Studying large-scale samples with various disease mechanisms using multiparametric imaging at function, structure and molecular scales, and revealing the correlations between the neuroimaging metrics and clinical data including neurocognitive function and neuropsychological inventories to elucidate multiple factors affecting the neurodegeneration processes in brain are of importance to disease diagnosis and treatment. There is an increasing body of literature which suggests that damage to the default mode network, hypothalamus, thalamus and hippocampus might been under-diagnosed and may account for some of the sequelae following the neurodegenerative injuries including mild traumatic brain injury and post-traumatic stress disorder. The neurobiology and some related imaging findings of four representative neurodegenerative diseases will be introduced and reviewed in this chapter, including brain region-specific and disease-related alterations, unique clinical symptom of each disease, as well as previous findings and challenges.

Chapter 2 – Resting-state functional MRI (RS-fMRI) has recently drawn much attention in detecting various robust neuronal functional connectivity patterns. The purpose of the present study was to identify neuronal network abnormalities connecting from several previously reviewed critical regions using advanced quantitative functional connectivity with MRI (fcMRI) based on RS-fMRI data in representative neurodegenerative patients compared to controls. Voxel-wise fractional amplitude of low frequency fluctuation (fALFF) method was also implemented to examine any local regional activity injuries.

Our fcMRI results support the concept that functional networks of default mode network (DMN), thalamic, hypothalamic and hippocampal connectivity, frontal and temporal cortical functional activity are involved in injury after MTBI or PTSD at variable degrees. And these imaging biomarkers may play a crucial role in elucidating the pathomechanisms of post concussion syndrome, dementia or stress disorder in these patients. Our results of disruption of functional hypothalamic connectivity and activity based on fALFF in patients with MTBI as well as significant correlations with post-concussion syndrome might help to resolve an array of clinical symptoms in MTBI related to sleep disturbance and fatigue. In PTSD patients, various abnormal functional activity and connectivities had been observed, including decreased DMN and hippocampal fcMRI but increased hypothalamic and ventromedial prefrontal (vmPFC) connectivity, and compensated cerebellar and occipital activities, but lower vmPFC, hippocampal and amygdala activities. MCI patients also had significantly lower fcMRI from the hippocampus and key memory regions such as medial prefrontal cortex, hypothalamus and posterior cingulate. The data also provided preliminary evidence of the potential usefulness of fcMRI analyses for the detection of abnormalities of functional coordination in MS. It had been demonstrated that the fcMRI patterns including DMN and thalamic connectivity as well as regional functional activity were altered in patients with MS, especially in the occipital and prefrontal regions. Such observations can increase the understanding of structural and functional deficits in MS. All the results in this study were consistent with previous findings, with some distinctive neuronal network differences found in each type of disease. Specific regional connectivity and activity patterns of neuronal networks and comprehensive applications will help to differentiate and diagnose more accurately each type of neurodegenerative diseases with various etiologies including traumatic accident and stress disorder, dementia and inflammation.

Chapter 3 – Since the interhemispheric functional integration plays an important role in communicating perceptual, cognitive, learning, attention and information processing, more detailed clinical data on neurodegenerative and psychiatric disorders regarding brain functional homotopy and systematic analyses are needed with further validation and application. Previous studies had shown good correspondence between homotopy imaging and myelin map. The purposes of this study are to: i. examine the functional homotopic differences in the four neurodegenerative diseases including PTSD, MTBI, MCI and MS compared to controls; ii. explore the correlations between quantitative VMHC values and various neurocognitive/neuropsychological tests in patients; and iii. validate with other metrics including structural connectivity and myelin map.

Regarding the VMHC differences, PTSD patients had lower homotopic connections in the parietal, temporal, thalamic radiation and optic radiation, subcortical striatum as well as frontal white matter areas, with very mild higher homotopic connections in the small regions of vmPFC compared to controls ($P < 0.01$). Different VMHC pattern of MTBI was found with patients showing lower VMHC values in the hippocampus, bilateral dorsolateral prefrontal, temporal and occipital cortices but higher VMHC in the vmPFC and small middle cingulate regions. On the other hand, MCI patients had lower homotopic connections in the cuneus and small middle frontal regions, but higher homotopic connections in the distributed temporal, occipital, motor and parietal cortices were observed ($P < 0.01$). In MS patients, significantly lower VMHC values were found mainly in the primary cortices compared with controls, including significant reductions of regional mean VMHC values in the primary visual, somatosensory, and motor cortices (all with $P < 0.04$) in MS, with increased VMHC in the subcortical areas, including the thalamus, insula, pallidum, and cerebellum.

In terms of imaging correlates of clinical tests, the regions that had lower homotopic values in PTSD patients were associated significantly with clinical symptoms. For instance, lower homotopic values in temporal and parietal cortices, thalamic radiation and optic radiation, and significant correlations of homotopic values in these regions with CAPS. Negative correlations were found between vmPFC homotopic value and GDS, ADAS and TICS in PTSD. Significant correlations between homotopic values in frontal, temporal, occipital and parietal regions and MMSE, AFQT total as well as sub-categories such as object and spatial cognitive functionality were found additionally. In MS patients, homotopic values in dorsolateral prefrontal, cerebellum and posterior cingulate were correlated positively with both fatigue and depression scores but at opposite directions. Multiple regional significant associations were found including homotopic values in visual, temporal, motor, frontal cortices and executive function, verbal fluency, information processing, working memory and attention, visual-perception, sustained attention and executive function. And finally, the VMHC values in several regions including cuneus, medial prefrontal and tempo-occipital conjunction areas correlated with MS EDSS score.

Chapter 4 –Previous studies had shown some preliminary results of white matter integrity deterioration and structural connectivity abnormalities in mild cognitive impairment (MCI), multiple sclerosis (MS), post traumatic stress disorder (PTSD) and mild traumatic brain injury (MTBI). In addition to identifying the functional network differences of the neurodegenerative diseases, the purposes of this study are to: i. investigate the microstructural DTI imaging and other morphological brain changes including volumetry under disease conditions; and ii. explore the graph-theory based small-worldness (SMW) differences in patients compared to controls of the four neurodegenerative diseases.

Microstructural FA metric identified disease-specific alterations in patients, including uncinate, major forceps, corticospinal and cingulum tracts deterioration in PTSD; significant fornix and hippocampal cingulum FA reduction in MCI; diffuse axonal injury in the frontal and occipital cortices and corpus callosum in MTBI; and lower FA in the corpus callosum and optic radiation in MS patients. In line with the abnormal micro-structure, molecular and functional imaging results, significant reductions of cortical thickness, surface area and volume involved in memory and executive function were found in PTSD and MCI patients, such as the pars opercularis, anterior cingulate, temporal pole and transverse temporal region in patients compared to controls. And finally the integrated small-worldness analyses showed similar characteristics in PTSD and AD/MCI patients, including local efficiency and small-worldness decreases but global efficiency increases. Despite no significant SMW differences in MS patients compared to controls, higher local efficiency but lower global efficiency in MTBI patients was identified additionally.

Chapter 5 –Some preliminary results of tau and amyloid imaging as well as neuroinflammation and metabolism dysfunction in PTSD, MTBI and MCI had been reported recently. In addition to identifying the functional and structural network differences of the neurodegenerative diseases, the purpose of this chapter is to quantify further available molecular imaging tracers such as tau, amyloid and FDG-glucose in the four neurodegenerative diseases.

The results showed significantly different molecular imaging patterns for distinguishing each neurodegenerative disease. In PTSD patients compared to controls, both regional quantification and Braak staging algorithm found significantly higher tau in the temporal, parietal and visual cortices such as hippocampus, anterior and posterior cingulate, precuneus and planum polare regions at stages II and later Braak stages VI, V and IV. While in MCI patients compared to controls, higher tau deposition was found in the early possible pathological regions of entorhinal, hippocampal and temporal cortices with significantly higher tau only in the early Braak stages I and II. Higher tau in the typical vmPFC and temporal region in PTSD patients in contrast to the higher tau in the thalamic/hypothalamic and orbitofrontal regions in TBI indicated different but overlapped neuropathological burdens of these two diseases. PTSD patients also had significantly higher amyloid accumulation in the temporal, occipital and inferior parietal lobes; while MCI patients showed higher degree of amyloid depositions both globally and regionally in the medial prefrontal and posterior cingulate cortices compared to controls. Different patterns of tau and amyloid depositions in MCI patients compared to PTSD/TBI and controls were exhibited, including higher tau at early Braak stages in MCI vs. much higher tau at later Braak stages in PTSD and higher at subcortical regions in TBI. Hypometabolism of glucose based on FDG PET imaging in PTSD and MCI patients compared to controls had been observed additionally. Our advanced neuroimaging quantifications including multiple molecular tracers demonstrated significant and distinct brain alterations at various scales in different types of neurodegenerative diseases with high sensitivity and specificity.

Chapter 6 – Previous studies including ours had demonstrated many applications of fcMRI in quantifying therapeutic effects, evaluating treatment efficacy such as traditional Chinese medicine (TCM) and implementation in other challenging diseases. The purposes of this study are to review some of the therapeutic effects of TCM with neuroimaging quantifications to help treating neurodegenerative diseases, and to summarize some imaging applications in other challenging diseases.

Chapter 7 – A summary of multiparametric imaging findings and correlations with clinical data in previous chapters 2-5 are listed in Tables in this Chapter. Some proposed and reviewed traditional Chinese medicines for neurodegenerative disease treatment in Chapter 6 are summarized in Table as well. A neurobiology model of the pathological processes such as accumulation of tau and amyloid (Aβ), demyelination and dysfunction in specific regions with the neurodegenerative diseases was proposed.

Chapter 1

INTRODUCTION AND APPLICATION OF NEUROIMAGING INCLUDING FUNCTIONAL NEURONAL NETWORK IN NEURODEGENERATIVE DISEASE

ABSTRACT

Studying large-scale samples with various disease mechanisms using multiparametric imaging at function, structure and molecular scales, as well as revealing the correlations between the neuroimaging metrics and clinical data including neurocognitive function and neuropsychological inventories to elucidate multiple factors affecting the neurodegeneration processes in brain are of importance to disease diagnosis and treatment. There is an increasing body of literature suggesting that damage to the default mode network, hypothalamus, thalamus and hippocampus might be under-diagnosed and may account for some of the sequelae following the neurodegenerative injuries including mild traumatic brain injury and post-traumatic stress disorder. The neurobiology and some related imaging findings of four representative neurodegenerative diseases will be introduced and reviewed in this chapter, including brain region-specific and disease-related alterations, unique clinical symptom of each disease, as well as previous findings and challenges.

INTRODUCTION

Applications of new imaging probes and correlating with other co-occurring functional and structural imaging findings together with biological data of injured brain and neurodegenerative disorder are of importance to improve early disease detection. Recent accumulating evidence indicates that each neuroimaging modality can provide unique imaging feature; and multiparametric imaging methods could help better interpret functional and structural changes in memory and dementia. Together with the clinical neurocognitive, neuropsychological and phenotypic data, these multiparametric metrics could innovate the research field of disease diagnosis and prevention. With the advanced multiple brain functional, structural and molecular imaging techniques, we can identify early neuroplastic and neuropathological changes in neurodegenerative diseases including early Alzheimer's disease (AD) [1, 2]. These rich advanced imaging features could provide specific disease-associated alterations and illustrate better the underlying pathological mechanism as well as improve diagnosis accuracy.

Studying large-scale samples with various disease mechanisms using multiparametric imaging, as well as revealing the correlations between the neuroimaging metrics and clinical data including neurocognitive function and neuropsychological inventories to elucidate multiple factors affecting the neurodegeneration processes in brain are the main topics of this book. In addition, the neural underpins of cognitive and psychological functions with advanced functional imaging techniques can provide better cross-validation and clinical symptom relevance of multiparametric data. Expanding the current findings with higher diagnosis accuracy and detection specificity in multiple neurodegenerative diseases as well as better differentiation of each type are the ultimate goal of our comprehensive project. The results in this book will extend the current notion of diagnosis value of various relatively new imaging techniques in multiple neurodegenerative diseases including traumatic brain injury (TBI), post-traumatic stress disorder (PTSD), multiple sclerosis (MS) and AD.

The neurobiology and some related imaging findings of four representative neurodegenerative diseases will be introduced and reviewed in this chapter, including brain region-specific and disease-related alterations, unique clinical symptom of each disease, as well as previous findings and challenges. There is an increasing body of literature suggesting that damage to the default mode network, hypothalamus, thalamus and hippocampus might be under-diagnosed and may account for some of the sequelae following the neurodegenerative injuries including trauma and dementia. The relatively novel imaging results to differentiate each disease with several neuronal networks and new imaging tracers will be presented in the rest of this book. Finally, our work prove that the multiparametric neuroimaging methods (about 12 metrics) and data in this book are the most forefront and up-to-date with enough sensitivity, precision and resolution.

REVIEW OF NEUROIMAGING IN NEURODEGENERATIVE DISEASES

Multiparametric neuroimaging techniques using well-developed and relatively new methods including functional, structural and molecular imaging will be used for the neurodegenerative disease detection and diagnosis in this book. These techniques include: a. functional connectivity based MRI (fcMRI) for neuronal network identification with four specific seed regions or regions of interest (ROIs) using resting-state fMRI (RS-fMRI) data. These multiple neuronal networks including seeds from default mode network (DMN), hypothalamus, thalamus and hippocampus that serve important roles in brain function and could provide clue to the underlying disease mechanisms. b. fractional amplitude of low frequency fluctuation (fALFF) for spontaneous brain activity or neuronal activation based on RS-fMRI data; c. functional voxel-mirrored homotopic correlation (VMHC) imaging for myelin-related conductivity and inter-hemispheric correlation based on RS-fMRI data; d. graph-theory based small-worldness (SMW) analysis using RS-fMRI; e. microstructural fractional anisotropy (FA) spatial statistics for white matter integrity based on MRI diffusion tensor imaging (DTI) technique; f. structural morphometry including volume, surface area and cortical thickness based on MRI structural data; and g. molecular imaging including amyloid, tau and FDG for neuropathological burdens quantification based on PET data. The imaging data such as VMHC imaging will further be correlated with the clinical data including neurocognitive tests in multiple domains (e.g., working memory, executive function, visual perception and attention, processing speed and accuracy) to reveal the neural manifestation of cognitive associations. Some other related work including recently-developed advanced neuroimaging techniques such as non-invasive voxel-wise fast simultaneous mapping of blood flow, oxygen extraction and metabolism, mesoscopic MRI relaxation parameter R2′ and integrated processing methods such as linear effects model had been reported in our previous studies [1-4].

To apply these imaging techniques, the neurobiology of the four representative neurodegenerative diseases including definitions, etiologies and symptoms, specific and unique brain regions and networks of injuries involved, as well as previous related imaging findings will be summarized in the next section for each disease.

a. Post-Traumatic Stress Disorder

Post-traumatic stress disorder (PTSD) is a psychiatric disorder characterized by intrusions or re-experiencing, avoidance, hyperarousal and negative alterations in cognition and mood, commonly caused by traumatic exposure to warfare, traffic accident or abuse (Diagnostic and Statistical Manual of Mental Disorders, DSM-V, 2013) [5]. Avoidance and numbing include efforts to avoid thoughts, feelings, conversations, activities, places, or people that arouse recollections of the trauma(s), inability to recall important aspects of the trauma(s), diminished interest in significant activities, feelings of detachment from others, restricted range of affect, and a sense of a foreshortened future (APA, 2000) [6]. Hyperarousal symptoms include difficulty falling asleep, irritability or anger, difficulty concentrating, hypervigilance, and an exaggerated startle response (APA, 2000) [7, 8]. These symptoms have been linked to deficits in episodic memory, attentional control, executive functions and working memory [9, 10].

In the brain, the hypothalamic–pituitary–adrenal (HPA) axis is a complex set of direct influences and feedback interactions between the hypothalamus, pituitary, and adrenal cortex [12, 13]. It is a major part of the neuroendocrine system that regulates and controls not only the response to stress but also many other bodily processes, such as digestion, metabolism, temperature regulation, mood, immune system function, sex drive, behavior, and cognitions [14-16]. The function of the HPA axis in response to stress is through the control and release of the human stress response hormone, cortisol. Under normal conditions, the hypothalamus releases corticotropin releasing hormone (CRH) and arginine vasopressin (AVP) from the hypothalamic paraventricular nucleus, circulating levels of cortisol and circadian rhythms [14, 17, 18]. On cellular level, the human lateral hypothalamus contains about 50,000-80,000 orexin neurons [19]. Orexin cell are located mainly in the lateral hypothalamus and have strong projections to the raphe nuclei (function of sleep/wake cycle), locus coeruleus (arousal, vigilance, stress response), tuberomammillary nucleus (arousal, sleep), orbito- and medial prefrontal cortices (function of arousal, attention) [19]. A relatively new family of neuropeptides, orexins or hypocretins, has been discovered to be integral in arousal, sleep/wake cycles, reward and motivation [20, 21]. Furthermore, activation of orexin neurons was also associated with a decreased arousal threshold (i.e., more prone to hyperarousal) and may play a role in the 'fight-or-flight' response to a threatening or stressful situation (e.g., avoidance) [22]. And it had been found that current treatments such as selective serotonin reuptake inhibitors and psychotherapy might have a beneficial impact on the HPA axis in PTSD populations [23].

PTSD is characterized by aberrant resting-state functional connectivity in multiple brain networks including the most robust DMN [24, 25]. For instance, fcMRI analyses revealed decreased DMN connectivity such as lower connectivity between posterior cingulate (PCC) and occipital cortex in patients compared to controls [26]. Moreover, within-DMN connectivity (between PCC and hippocampus) correlated negatively with symptom dimensions (severity and anxiety), while increased between-network connectivity including the DMN-salience network (SN) [27] and DMN-central executive network (CEN) [28] correlated positively with episodic memory measures. Decreased within-DMN connectivity and disrupted DMN-SN and DMN-CEN coupling could form the basis for intrusive trauma recollection and impaired episodic autobiographical recall in PTSD [26]. In addition, decreased connectivity between amygdala and dorsolateral prefrontal cortex, anterior cingulated cortex (ACC), and anterior insula correlated with depression symptom severity. Furthermore, elevated connectivity between the amygdala and the ventromedial prefrontal cortex (vmPFC) correlated with anxiety symptom severity [29]. Deficits in emotion regulation function due to hyperactive and hyperconnected SN and its hypoconnectivity with lateral prefrontal regions are thought to underlie the hyperarousal symptoms of PTSD [7, 30]. vmPFC is one of the key regions involved in PTSD that plays important roles in processing of fear and risk, as well as social morality; and has afferent connection with amygdala that regulates emotion including fears, anxiety, depression and pain [29]. Increased fcMRI between the left superior colliculus (SC) and the right dorsolateral prefrontal cortex as well as between the right SC and the right temporo-parietal junction paralleled the unique symptom profile and defensive responses observed in PTSD together with its dissociate subtype. Revealing brain changes in PTSD caused by different injury mechanisms could provide therapeutic guidance to the disease [31].

The hippocampus, one of the key regions in memory system, not only provides inhibition to HPA axis activation but also plays a vital role in learning new information [32].

Task-based fMRI studies have suggested abnormal functioning in regions implicated in attention and working memory [33] as well as memory representation [34] in PTSD, such as the medial temporal and posterior brain regions including hippocampal, parietal, and occipital areas. As reported, the mean left hippocampal volume for the torture-related (TR)-PTSD group was significantly lower than the healthy volunteer group [25].

Magnetoencephalography (MEG) contrasts of the neurophysiological networks involving in the processing of angry in contrast to happy faces showed that the PTSD group had elevated oscillatory connectivity for angry faces [35]. Maladaptive hyper-synchrony in PTSD for threatening faces was seen in subcortical regions including the thalamus, as well as cortical vmPFC, cingulum, inferior temporal and parietal regions. The benzodiazepine receptor ligand [123I]-iomazenil was studied and results found decreased prefrontal cortical binding in veterans with PTSD [25].

Furthermore, several studies used MRI/MRS to show smaller volume of the hippocampus and/or reduced neuronal activation in the hippocampus, a brain area that mediates verbal declarative memory in PTSD [36-38]. One of the possible pathomechanisms was that prolonged stress, together with cortisol hypersecretions, could cause hippocampal atrophy in PTSD. Cognitive deficits, such as memory impairments and poor performance of attentional tasks, have been found in samples of veterans [39], violence-related victims [40], abuse-related patients [41], children, pregnant women and adolescents with PTSD [42-44]. For combat-related PTSD, the clinical manifestations included not only intrusive recurrent memories and hypervigilance but also nonspecific symptoms such as insomnia, concentration difficulties, irritability, impaired decision-making abilities, and memory problems [42]. Taken together, multiple networks including vmPFC, hypothalamus, DMN and hippocampus might be damaged in PTSD patients and could be associated with the post-traumatic symptoms. Systematic multiparametric imaging results using functional, homotopy, microstructural, morphological, and molecular metrics have not been reported previously.

b. Mild Traumatic Brain Injury

Mild traumatic brain injury (MTBI) is a significant public health problem, representing 75% of the total TBI cases. However, its underlying pathophysiological mechanisms of complex posttraumatic symptoms are poorly understood, leading to a paucity of successful treatment strategies [45]. There is usually no evidence of brain structural abnormality on conventional neuroimaging, such as CT and MRI scans [46]. There are quite a few recently developed advanced neuroimaging techniques including fMRI for detecting brain abnormalities in MTBI such as DMN dysfunction, thalamic and hypothalamic injury, disruption of thalamo-cortical connections as well as long-term white matter atrophies [1, 47-50]. In MTBI, Mayer and colleagues had also found abnormal connectivity between the DMN and frontal cortex [51]. Furthermore, there is increasing evidence of functional disconnectivity between deep gray matter and cortex including basal ganglia and thalamus as well as lower neuronal activity [47, 48]. In TBI, diffuse axonal injury resulting in disruption of functional networks in the brain is thought to be a major contributor to cognitive dysfunction in survivors of traumatic brain injury [52]. Following brain injury, there is significant disruption or decreased fcMRI between brain regions in patients with TBI [53]. Either hypometabolism at DMN or hyper-connectivity in the frontal regions had been reported in patients with diffuse axonal injury, chronic TBI or vegetative conditions [54-56].

The thalamus has been described as the anatomic threshold to consciousness [57]. It is the central relay station of the brain and is also an important and primary generator of brain waves such as alpha (with frequency between 8 to 12 Hz) and gamma waves (with frequency between 25 to 100 Hz) [48]. Alpha waves are associated with relaxed awareness in an idle state [58-60]. On the other hand, gamma waves are associated with conscious perception and play a role in the interaction and organization of multimodality inputs (e.g., motor and sensory) [61, 62]. On a cellular level, recent findings on pacemaker neurons suggest that these thalamic spindles could lead to synchronized cortical network oscillations within the gamma band by entraining other cells with their firing patterns [60]. One of the suggested mechanisms for conscious attention of the gamma wave originating in the thalamus and its importance for conscious awareness under coma situation had been proposed by Pollack [63]. He goes on to say that "If the thalamus was damaged even a little bit", such as in traumatic episode case, "the gamma wave stops, conscious awareness do not form, and the patient slips into profound coma". Likewise, if the coupling between the thalamus and other brain structures is hindered, the impact of arousal related processes on cerebral responses may become impaired [64, 65]. And in the resting state, another important function of the thalamic reticular nuclei is the inhibition. These nuclei have rich g-aminobutyric acid (GABA)-ergic neurons, which act as inhibitory intermediaries not only within thalamic nuclei but also for longer-range thalamo-cortical interaction [66, 67].

It is well known that orexin/hypocretin increases the craving for food, and correlates with the function of the substances that promote its production since hypocretin is recently found to be a very important link that integrates metabolism and sleep regulation [21]. Studies including ours have suggested that hypothalamus plays a key role in appetite regulation and lesions to the hypothalamus might change the visual perception of food and related neuronal circuits [1, 20, 68]. Orexin neurons regulate sleep, wakefulness and the maintenance of wakefulness through excitatory projections to the entire central nervous system (CNS) (excluding the cerebellum) with particularly dense projections to nuclei in the brain stem and hypothalamic regions. Orexin neurons also have links with the reward system through the ventral tegmental area (VTA) and with the hypothalamic nuclei that stimulate feeding behavior [69]. Orexin neuropeptide has been shown to increase wakefulness by decreasing non-rapid eye movement (REM) and REM sleep; and orexin neurons increase firing during wakefulness and decrease during slow wave sleep and twitch-free REM. It had been reported that low cerebrospinal fluid (CSF) levels of orexin and orexin receptor knockout mice/rats were associated with narcolepsy with cataplexy [19, 70].

The commonly reported sequelae following TBI of any severity include fatigue, problems with sleep, problems with appetite and arousal, and lack of motivation [71], which are all closely related to hypothalamic dysfunction and neuropeptide dysregulation [72]. There is an increasing body of literature indicating that damage to the HPA has been under-diagnosed and may account for some of the sequelae following TBI of any severity [73]. In MTBI, these sequelae may be reported immediately but in some cases (up to 30%) can develop and persist months to years after the injury [49, 74]. While damage following moderate to severe TBI can be easily envisioned, MTBI can also cause injury to hypothalamic cell bodies that may result in substantial neuropeptide dysregulation with associated clinical hypothalamic symptoms related to motivated behavior, sleep/wake cycles, and arousal [19, 72]. However, there are few studies investigating the hypothalamic injury in MTBI in vivo and its role in post concussion syndrome is largely underappreciated.

Our recent results demonstrated lower posterior DMN functional connectivity with compensated higher anterior DMN connectivity in MTBI patients compared to controls, as well as lower neuronal activity and functional connectivity in the thalamus and hypothalamus, disruption of thalamo-cortical connections and hypothalamic fcMRI in patients [1, 47, 48]. Our recent study also found disruption of functional and microstructural hypothalamic connectivity MTBI, and significant correlation with the fatigue severity scale, which might further the understanding of an array of clinical symptoms in MTBI such as sleep disturbance and fatigue. In addition, significant functional small-world properties changes in patients with MTBI had been reported with decreased global efficiency that was possibly due to diffuse axonal injury or white matter atrophy, and local network upregulation such as increased thalamo-cortical connectivity after injury [49, 75]. Having some similar injury mechanism as PTSD, the neuropathological burdens such as tau, amyloid and demyelination or other brain changes have not been studied extensively in MTBI.

c. Mild Cognitive Impairment

Identifying distinctive biomarkers of functional imaging in the early stage of Alzheimer's Disease (AD) and the prodrome of dementia, such as mild cognitive impairment (MCI), might provide opportunities for intervention and could delay the onset of the clinical manifestations of dementia [76, 77]. One of the hallmarks of AD is amyloid pathology within the cerebral cortex accompanied by cortical thinning, structural reorganization, and recruitment of new areas for functional adaptation at early or preclinical stages of disease including MCI [78, 79]. The earliest neuropathologic changes including amyloid plaques and tau tangles associated with MCI/AD occur in the entorhinal and hippocampal cortices [80, 81].

Our recent studies confirmed that primary age-related tauopahty occurred mainly in the temporal cortex including the hippocampus; and longitudinal changes of intracellular tau tangles were mostly accumulated in the temporal pole and middle temporal cortex at preclinical stage [2, 81]. Recent research suggests abnormal metabolic and hemodynamic changes in MCI/AD occur predominantly in the PCC, medial temporal lobe (MTL), and inferior parietal lobe (IPL) [82, 83]. Our previous study of fMRI and diffusion tensor imaging (DTI) data confirmed decreased functional and structural connectivities from both the PCC and hippocampus to the whole brain in MCI and AD patients, as well as reduction in connectivity between these two regions [76].

Another our study of the RS-fMRI results found reduced functional connectivity in the DMN medial prefrontal cortex (MPFC) region and reduced functional activity by means of fALFF in the temporal region in MCI patients compared with controls [84]. The fALFF activity was also reduced in temporal region in AD compared with MCI patients, but increased in the parietal region. Although being one of the most representative and extensively studied aging-related diseases, the detailed comparisons of multiparametric imaging between MCI/AD and other neurodegenerative diseases have not been analyzed comprehensively.

d. Multiple Sclerosis

Multiple sclerosis (MS) is a chronic inflammatory demyelinating disease that affects the whole brain. Neuroimaging techniques that can help elucidate and characterize the nature and mechanism of tissue injury and disease progression in MS are of particular importance given its roles in seeking successful preventive and therapeutic treatments of the disease [85-87]. Imaging biomarkers include multiple lesions, brain atrophy and normal appearing brain tissue abnormalities [88-90]. Although MS is considered to be an autoimmune inflammatory disease that primarily activates hematogenous macrophages that destroy myelin, growing evidence strongly suggests that MS is a diffuse neurodegenerative disease. Using RS-fMRI and DTI [49, 91-93], several studies had reported functional and structural connectivity impairments in patients including networks of sensorimotor and visual cortices in MS [94, 95]. For instance, decreased functional connectivity in MS patients [96] and increased inter-hemispheric strengths of coefficients of effective connectivity in MS were reported [97, 98]. These studies, however, all focused on a specific functional pathway. Our group had recently reported the changes of interhemispheric functional connectivity (i.e., voxel mirrored homotopic correlation, VMHC) and associated reduced FA in corpus callosum (CC) in patients [87]. And we also found cerebrovascular reactivity deficits in MS based on blood flow and neuronal activation measured with fMRI [99]. Abnormalities of other functional connectivity networks in MS including fcMRI from hypothalamus and hippocampus as well as functional activity with more advanced imaging techniques and association with clinical symptoms need to be examined further [100].

References

[1] Zhou Y. *Neuroimaging in Multiple Sclerosis.* Nova Science Publishers 2017.

[2] Zhou Y. *Function and Metabolism of Aging: Longitudinal Neuroimaging Evaluation.* Nova Science Publishers 2019.

[3] Zhou Y. *Functional Neuroimaging with Multiple Modalities: Principles, Devices and Applications.* Nova Science Publishers 2016.

[4] Zhou Y. *Neuroimaging in Mild Traumatic Brain Injury.* Nova Science Publishers 2017.

[5] Dean KR, Hammamieh R, Mellon SH, et al. Multi-omic biomarker identification and validation for diagnosing warzone-related post-traumatic stress disorder. *Mol Psychiatry* 2019.

[6] Jones T, Moller MD. Implications of hypothalamic-pituitary-adrenal axis functioning in posttraumatic stress disorder. *J Am Psychiatr Nurses Assoc* 2011;17:393-403.

[7] Lanius RA, Bluhm R, Lanius U, Pain C. A review of neuroimaging studies in PTSD: heterogeneity of response to symptom provocation. *J Psychiatr Res* 2006;40:709-729.

[8] Van Boven RW, Harrington GS, Hackney DB, et al. Advances in neuroimaging of traumatic brain injury and posttraumatic stress disorder. *J Rehabil Res Dev* 2009;46:717-757.

[9] Kavanaugh BC, Dupont-Frechette JA, Jerskey BA, Holler KA. Neurocognitive deficits in children and adolescents following maltreatment: Neurodevelopmental consequences and neuropsychological implications of traumatic stress. *Appl Neuropsychol Child* 2017;6:64-78.

[10] Scott JC, Matt GE, Wrocklage KM, et al. A quantitative meta-analysis of neurocognitive functioning in posttraumatic stress disorder. *Psychol Bull* 2015;141:105-140.

[11] Rangaprakash D, Deshpande G, Daniel TA, et al. Compromised hippocampus-striatum pathway as a potential imaging biomarker of mild-traumatic brain injury and posttraumatic stress disorder. *Hum Brain Mapp* 2017;38:2843-2864.

[12] Jones EJ. *The Thalamus.* Cambridge University Press; 2 edition 2007;2.

[13] Hoffman AN, Taylor AN. Stress reactivity after traumatic brain injury: implications for comorbid post-traumatic stress disorder. *Behav Pharmacol* 2019;30:115-121.

[14] Felmingham K, Williams LM, Whitford TJ, et al. Duration of posttraumatic stress disorder predicts hippocampal grey matter loss. *Neuroreport* 2009;20:1402-1406.

[15] Higgins ES, Kose S. Absence of schizophrenia in a 15th-century Islamic medical textbook. *Am J Psychiatry* 2007;164:1120; author reply 1120-1121.

[16] Matus-Amat P, Higgins EA, Sprunger D, Wright-Hardesty K, Rudy JW. The role of dorsal hippocampus and basolateral amygdala NMDA receptors in the acquisition and retrieval of context and contextual fear memories. *Behav Neurosci* 2007;121:721-731.

[17] Clifford RE, Baker D, Risbrough VB, Huang M, Yurgil KA. Impact of TBI, PTSD, and Hearing Loss on Tinnitus Progression in a US Marine Cohort. *Mil Med* 2019.

[18] Jackson S, Baity MR, Bobb K, Swick D, Giorgio J. Stress inoculation training outcomes among veterans with PTSD and TBI. *Psychol Trauma* 2019.

[19] Nunez A, Rodrigo-Angulo ML, Andres ID, Garzon M. Hypocretin/ Orexin neuropeptides: participation in the control of sleep-wakefulness cycle and energy homeostasis. *Curr Neuropharmacol* 2009;7:50-59.

[20] de Lecea L, Kilduff TS, Peyron C, et al. The hypocretins: hypothalamus-specific peptides with neuroexcitatory activity. *Proc Natl Acad Sci U S A* 1998;95:322-327.

[21] Sakurai T, Amemiya A, Ishii M, et al. Orexins and orexin receptors: a family of hypothalamic neuropeptides and G protein-coupled receptors that regulate feeding behavior. *Cell* 1998;92:1 page following 696.

[22] Adamantidis A, de Lecea L. The hypocretins as sensors for metabolism and arousal. *J Physiol* 2009;587:33-40.

[23] Polusny MA, Kehle SM, Nelson NW, Erbes CR, Arbisi PA, Thuras P. Longitudinal effects of mild traumatic brain injury and

posttraumatic stress disorder comorbidity on postdeployment outcomes in national guard soldiers deployed to Iraq. *Arch Gen Psychiatry* 2011;68:79-89.

[24] Fu S, Ma X, Wu Y, et al. Altered Local and Large-Scale Dynamic Functional Connectivity Variability in Posttraumatic Stress Disorder: A Resting-State fMRI Study. *Front Psychiatry* 2019;10:234.

[25] Zandieh S, Bernt R, Knoll P, et al. Analysis of the Metabolic and Structural Brain Changes in Patients With Torture-Related Post-Traumatic Stress Disorder (TR-PTSD) Using (1)(8)F-FDG PET and MRI. *Medicine (Baltimore)* 2016;95:e3387.

[26] Viard A, Mutlu J, Chanraud S, et al. Altered default mode network connectivity in adolescents with post-traumatic stress disorder. *Neuroimage Clin* 2019;22:101731.

[27] Jack CR, Jr., Knopman DS, Jagust WJ, et al. Tracking pathophysiological processes in Alzheimer's disease: an updated hypothetical model of dynamic biomarkers. *Lancet Neurol* 2013; 12:207-216.

[28] Zhou J, Jaquet A, Bissagnene E, et al. Short-term risk of anaemia following initiation of combination antiretroviral treatment in HIV-infected patients in countries in sub-Saharan Africa, Asia-Pacific, and central and South America. *J Int AIDS Soc* 2012;15:5.

[29] Corcoran KA, Quirk GJ. Recalling safety: cooperative functions of the ventromedial prefrontal cortex and the hippocampus in extinction. *CNS Spectr* 2007;12:200-206.

[30] Fonzo GA, Simmons AN, Thorp SR, Norman SB, Paulus MP, Stein MB. Exaggerated and disconnected insular-amygdalar blood oxygenation level-dependent response to threat-related emotional faces in women with intimate-partner violence posttraumatic stress disorder. *Biol Psychiatry* 2010;68:433-441.

[31] Olive I, Densmore M, Harricharan S, Theberge J, McKinnon MC, Lanius R. Superior colliculus resting state networks in post-traumatic stress disorder and its dissociative subtype. *Hum Brain Mapp* 2018;39:563-574.

[32] Zhou Y, Shu N, Liu Y, et al. Altered resting-state functional connectivity and anatomical connectivity of hippocampus in schizophrenia. *Schizophr Res* 2008;100:120-132.

[33] Aupperle RL, Melrose AJ, Stein MB, Paulus MP. Executive function and PTSD: disengaging from trauma. *Neuropharmacology* 2012;62:686-694.

[34] Lazarov A, Zhu X, Suarez-Jimenez B, Rutherford BR, Neria Y. Resting-state functional connectivity of anterior and posterior hippocampus in posttraumatic stress disorder. *J Psychiatr Res* 2017;94:15-22.

[35] Dunkley BT, Wong SM, Jetly R, Wong JK, Taylor MJ. Post-traumatic stress disorder and chronic hyperconnectivity in emotional processing. *Neuroimage Clin* 2018;20:197-204.

[36] Astur RS, St Germain SA, Tolin D, Ford J, Russell D, Stevens M. Hippocampus function predicts severity of post-traumatic stress disorder. *Cyberpsychol Behav* 2006;9:234-240.

[37] Smith ME. Bilateral hippocampal volume reduction in adults with post-traumatic stress disorder: a meta-analysis of structural MRI studies. *Hippocampus* 2005;15:798-807.

[38] Friedman MJ, Resick PA, Bryant RA, Brewin CR. Considering PTSD for DSM-V. *Depress Anxiety* 2011;28:750-769.

[39] Vasterling JJ, Duke LM, Brailey K, Constans JI, Allain AN, Jr., Sutker PB. Attention, learning, and memory performances and intellectual resources in Vietnam veterans: PTSD and no disorder comparisons. *Neuropsychology* 2002;16:5-14.

[40] Jenkins MA, Langlais PJ, Delis D, Cohen R. Learning and memory in rape victims with posttraumatic stress disorder. *Am J Psychiatry* 1998;155:278-279.

[41] Elzinga BM, Schmahl CG, Vermetten E, van Dyck R, Bremner JD. Higher cortisol levels following exposure to traumatic reminders in abuse-related PTSD. *Neuropsychopharmacology* 2003;28:1656-1665.

[42] Bremner JD, Vythilingam M, Vermetten E, et al. Cortisol response to a cognitive stress challenge in posttraumatic stress disorder

(PTSD) related to childhood abuse. *Psychoneuroendocrinology* 2003;28:733-750.

[43] Moradi AR, Taghavi MR, Neshat Doost HT, Yule W, Dalgleish T. Performance of children and adolescents with PTSD on the Stroop colour-naming task. *Psychol Med* 1999;29:415-419.

[44] Lopez WD, Seng JS. Posttraumatic stress disorder, smoking, and cortisol in a community sample of pregnant women. *Addict Behav* 2014;39:1408-1413.

[45] Silver JM, McAllister TW, Yudofsky SC. *Textbook of Traumatic Brain Injury.* American Psychiatric Publishing, Inc. 2011;2nd Edition.

[46] Jantzen KJ. Functional magnetic resonance imaging of mild traumatic brain injury. *J Head Trauma Rehabil* 2010;25:256-266.

[47] Zhou Y, Milham MP, Lui YW, et al. Default-mode network disruption in mild traumatic brain injury. *Radiology* 2012;265:882-892.

[48] Zhou Y, Lui YW, Zuo XN, et al. Characterization of thalamo-cortical association using amplitude and connectivity of functional MRI in mild traumatic brain injury. *J Magn Reson Imaging* 2014;39:1558-1568.

[49] Zhou Y, Kierans A, Kenul D, et al. Mild traumatic brain injury: longitudinal regional brain volume changes. *Radiology* 2013;267:880-890.

[50] Zhou Y. *Traumatic Brain Injury: Neurbiology, Diagnosis and Treatment.* Editor, Intechopen Publisher 2019.

[51] Mayer AR, Mannell MV, Ling J, Gasparovic C, Yeo RA. Functional connectivity in mild traumatic brain injury. *Hum Brain Mapp* 2011.

[52] Smith DH, Meaney DF, Shull WH. Diffuse axonal injury in head trauma. *J Head Trauma Rehabil* 2003;18:307-316.

[53] Hillary FG, Slocomb J, Hills EC, et al. Changes in resting connectivity during recovery from severe traumatic brain injury. *Int J Psychophysiol* 2011.

[54] Cauda F, Micon BM, Sacco K, et al. Disrupted intrinsic functional connectivity in the vegetative state. *J Neurol Neurosurg Psychiatry* 2009;80:429-431.

[55] Kim J, Whyte J, Patel S, et al. Resting cerebral blood flow alterations in chronic traumatic brain injury: an arterial spin labeling perfusion FMRI study. *J Neurotrauma* 2010;27:1399-1411.

[56] Nakashima T, Nakayama N, Miwa K, Okumura A, Soeda A, Iwama T. Focal brain glucose hypometabolism in patients with neuropsychologic deficits after diffuse axonal injury. *AJNR Am J Neuroradiol* 2007;28:236-242.

[57] Jones EJ. The Thalamus. Cambridge University Press; 2 edition 2007;2.

[58] Chatila M, Milleret C, Rougeul A, Buser P. Alpha rhythm in the cat thalamus. *C R Acad Sci III* 1993;316:51-58.

[59] Lopes da Silva FH, Hoeks A, Smits H, Zetterberg LH. Model of brain rhythmic activity. The alpha-rhythm of the thalamus. *Kybernetik* 1974;15:27-37.

[60] Schreckenberger M, Lange-Asschenfeldt C, Lochmann M, et al. The thalamus as the generator and modulator of EEG alpha rhythm: a combined PET/EEG study with lorazepam challenge in humans. *Neuroimage* 2004;22:637-644.

[61] Buzsaki G, Wang XJ. Mechanisms of gamma oscillations. *Annu Rev Neurosci* 2012;35:203-225.

[62] Engel AK, Fries P, Konig P, Brecht M, Singer W. Temporal binding, binocular rivalry, and consciousness. *Conscious Cogn* 1999;8:128-151.

[63] Pollack R. *The Missing Moment: How the Unconscious Shapes Modern Science.* Houghton Mifflin 1999.

[64] Kempf F, Brucke C, Salih F, et al. Gamma activity and reactivity in human thalamic local field potentials. *Eur J Neurosci* 2009;29:943-953.

[65] Sun Y, Farzan F, Barr MS, et al. gamma oscillations in schizophrenia: mechanisms and clinical significance. *Brain Res* 2011;1413:98-114.

[66] Aron AR, Schlaghecken F, Fletcher PC, et al. Inhibition of subliminally primed responses is mediated by the caudate and thalamus: evidence from functional MRI and Huntington's disease. *Brain* 2003;126:713-723.
[67] Steriade M. Sleep, epilepsy and thalamic reticular inhibitory neurons. *Trends Neurosci* 2005;28:317-324.
[68] Zhou Y. Abnormal structural and functional hypothalamic connectivity in mild traumatic brain injury. J Magn Reson Imaging 2017;45:1105-1112.
[69] Sakurai T. The neural circuit of orexin (hypocretin): maintaining sleep and wakefulness. *Nat Rev Neurosci* 2007;8:171-181.
[70] Bourgin P, Zeitzer JM, Mignot E. CSF hypocretin-1 assessment in sleep and neurological disorders. *Lancet Neurol* 2008;7:649-662.
[71] Castriotta RJ, Wilde MC, Lai JM, Atanasov S, Masel BE, Kuna ST. Prevalence and consequences of sleep disorders in traumatic brain injury. *J Clin Sleep Med* 2007;3:349-356.
[72] Baumann CR, Werth E, Stocker R, Ludwig S, Bassetti CL. Sleep-wake disturbances 6 months after traumatic brain injury: a prospective study. *Brain* 2007;130:1873-1883.
[73] Haacke EM, Xu Y, Cheng YC, Reichenbach JR. Susceptibility weighted imaging (SWI). *Magn Reson Med* 2004;52:612-618.
[74] Petchprapai N, Winkelman C. Mild traumatic brain injury: determinants and subsequent quality of life. A review of the literature. *J Neurosci Nurs* 2007;39:260-272.
[75] Zhou Y. Small world properties changes in mild traumatic brain injury. *J Magn Reson Imaging* 2017;46:518-527.
[76] Zhou Y, Dougherty JH, Jr., Hubner KF, Bai B, Cannon RL, Hutson RK. Abnormal connectivity in the posterior cingulate and hippocampus in early Alzheimer's disease and mild cognitive impairment. *Alzheimers Dement* 2008;4:265-270.
[77] Zhou Y, Lui YW. Small-World Properties in Mild Cognitive Impairment and Early Alzheimer's Disease: A Cortical Thickness MRI Study. *ISRN Geriatr* 2013; 542080.

[78] Drzezga A, Becker JA, Van Dijk KRA, et al. Neuronal dysfunction and disconnection of cortical hubs in non-demented subjects with elevated amyloid burden. *Brain* 2011.

[79] Greicius MD, Krasnow B, Reiss AL, Menon V. Functional connectivity in the resting brain: a network analysis of the default mode hypothesis. *Proc Natl Aca Sci U S A* 2004;101:4637-4642.

[80] Sperling R, Mormino E, Johnson K. The evolution of preclinical Alzheimer's disease: implications for prevention trials. *Neuron* 2014;84:608-622.

[81] Zhou Y, Bai B. Tau and Pet/Mri Imaging Biomarkers for Detecting and Diagnosing Early Dementia. Jacobs J Med Diagn Med Imaging 2017;2.

[82] Buckner RL, Snyder AZ, Shannon BJ, et al. Molecular, structural, and functional characterization of Alzheimer's disease: evidence for a relationship between default activity, amyloid, and memory. *J Neurosci* 2005;25:7709-7717.

[83] Raichle ME, Snyder AZ. A default mode of brain function: a brief history of an evolving idea. *Neuroimage* 2007;37:1083-1090; discussion 1097-1089.

[84] Zhou Y, Yu F, Duong TQ, Alzheimer's Disease Neuroimaging I. White matter lesion load is associated with resting state functional MRI activity and amyloid PET but not FDG in mild cognitive impairment and early Alzheimer's disease patients. *J Magn Reson Imaging* 2015;41:102-109.

[85] Trapp BD, Nave KA. Multiple sclerosis: an immune or neurodegenerative disorder? *Annu Rev Neurosci* 2008;31:247-269.

[86] Trapp BD, Ransohoff R, Rudick R. Axonal pathology in multiple sclerosis: relationship to neurologic disability. *Curr Opin Neurol* 1999;12:295-302.

[87] Zhou Y, Milham M, Zuo XN, et al. Functional Homotopic Changes in Multiple Sclerosis with Resting-State Functional MR Imaging. *AJNR Am J Neuroradiol* 2013.

[88] Lisak RP. Neurodegeneration in multiple sclerosis: defining the problem. *Neurology* 2007;68:S5-12; discussion S43-54.

[89] Prineas JW, McDonald WI. Demyelinating diseases. In: Graham DI, Lantos PL, eds. *Greenfield's Neuropathology*. London: Oxford University Press, 1997: 813-896.

[90] Rocca MA, Filippi M. Functional MRI in multiple sclerosis. *J Neuroimaging* 2007;17 Suppl 1:36S-41S.

[91] Zivadinov R, Cox JL. Neuroimaging in multiple sclerosis. *Int Rev Neurobiol* 2007;79:449-474.

[92] Zivadinov R, Ramasamy DP, Vaneckova M, et al. Leptomeningeal contrast enhancement is associated with progression of cortical atrophy in MS: A retrospective, pilot, observational longitudinal study. *Mult Scler* 2016.

[93] Smith SM, Jenkinson M, Johansen-Berg H, et al. Tract-based spatial statistics: voxelwise analysis of multi-subject diffusion data. *Neuroimage* 2006;31:1487-1505.

[94] Forn C, Barros-Loscertales A, Escudero J, et al. Compensatory activations in patients with multiple sclerosis during preserved performance on the auditory N-back task. *Hum Brain Mapp* 2007;28:424-430.

[95] Rocca MA, De Meo E, Filippi M. Functional MRI in investigating cognitive impairment in multiple sclerosis. *Acta Neurol Scand* 2016;134 Suppl 200:39-46.

[96] Lowe MJ, Beall EB, Sakaie KE, et al. Resting state sensorimotor functional connectivity in multiple sclerosis inversely correlates with transcallosal motor pathway transverse diffusivity. *Hum Brain Mapp* 2008;29:818-827.

[97] Rocca MA, Preziosa P, Mesaros S, et al. Clinically Isolated Syndrome Suggestive of Multiple Sclerosis: Dynamic Patterns of Gray and White Matter Changes-A 2-year MR Imaging Study. *Radiology* 2016;278:841-853.

[98] Rocca MA, Vacchi L, Rodegher M, et al. Mapping face encoding using functional MRI in multiple sclerosis across disease phenotypes. *Brain Imaging Behav* 2016.

[99] Zhou Y, Rodgers ZB, Kuo AH. Cerebrovascular reactivity measured with arterial spin labeling and blood oxygen level dependent techniques. *Magn Reson Imaging* 2015;33:566-576.

[100] Zhou Y. *Functional Neuroimaging Methods and Frontiers*. Nova Science Publishers 2018.

Chapter 2

ABNORMAL FUNCTIONAL CONNECTIVITY NETWORK IN MILD TRAUMATIC BRAIN INJURY, POST-TRAUMATIC STRESS DISORDER, MILD COGNITIVE IMPAIRMENT AND MULTIPLE SCLEROSIS

ABSTRACT

Resting-state functional MRI (RS-fMRI) has recently drawn much attention in detecting various robust neuronal functional connectivity patterns. The purpose of the present study was to identify neuronal network abnormalities connecting from several previously reviewed critical regions using advanced quantitative functional connectivity with MRI (fcMRI) based on RS-fMRI data in representative neurodegenerative patients compared to controls. Voxel-wise fractional amplitude of low frequency fluctuation (fALFF) method was also implemented to examine any local regional activity injuries.

Our fcMRI results support the concept that functional networks of default mode network (DMN), thalamic, hypothalamic and hippocampal connectivity, frontal and temporal cortical functional activity are involved in injury after mild traumatic brain injury (MTBI) or post-traumatic stress disorder (PTSD) at variable degrees. And these imaging biomarkers may play a crucial role in elucidating the pathomechanisms of post concussion syndrome, dementia or stress disorder in these patients. Our results of disruption of functional hypothalamic connectivity and activity based on fALFF in patients with MTBI as well as significant correlations with post-concussion syndrome might help to resolve an array of clinical symptoms in MTBI related to sleep disturbance and fatigue. In PTSD patients, various abnormal functional activity and connectivities had been observed, including decreased DMN and hippocampal fcMRI but increased hypothalamic and ventromedial prefrontal cortex (vmPFC) connectivity, and compensated cerebellar and occipital activities, but lower vmPFC, hippocampal and amygdala activities. Mild cognitive impairment (MCI) patients also had significantly lower fcMRI from the hippocampus and key memory regions such as medial prefrontal cortex, hypothalamus and posterior cingulate. The data also provided preliminary evidence of the potential usefulness of fcMRI analyses for the detection of abnormalities of functional coordination in multiple sclerosis (MS). It had been demonstrated that the fcMRI patterns including DMN and thalamic connectivity as well as regional functional activity were altered in patients with MS, especially in the occipital and prefrontal regions. Such observations can increase the understanding of structural and functional deficits in MS. All the results in this study were consistent with previous findings, with some distinctive neuronal network differences found in each type of disease. Specific regional connectivity and activity patterns of neuronal networks and comprehensive applications will help to differentiate and diagnose more accurately each type of neurodegenerative diseases with various etiologies including traumatic accident and stress disorder, dementia and inflammation.

INTRODUCTION

Using functional connectivity with MRI (fcMRI), critical brain networks can be evaluated without performing a particular task [1]. Resting state (RS)-fMRI has recently drawn more attention in detecting various robust neuronal functional connectivity patterns [2]. Based on RS-fMRI data, studies have consistently demonstrated phase-locked low-frequency oscillations (< 0.1 Hz) of blood oxygen level-dependent (BOLD) signal across functionally connected brain regions (resting state networks, RSNs) in the resting brain [3, 4]. There are several well-established intrinsic brain networks at resting state including default mode network (DMN) [5], the anti-DMN dorsal attention network (DAN) [6], central executive network [7], sensorimotor and visual networks [8]. These RSNs were characterized by highly correlated time courses of robust low-frequency fluctuation signals across functional connected regions, which reflect underlying neuronal synchronous firing [3]. DMN is the most robust and well-studied network, and brain regions involved are of pivotal importance to daily life [4]. These brain nodes form a functional entity including the hippocampus and posterior cingulate cortex (PCC) for memory encoding, consolidation and retrieval, and for environmental monitoring, as well as medial prefrontal cortex (MPFC) for higher-order cognitive and social functions such as self-relevance, rapid error identification, and communication functions [3, 9-12]. Brain neuronal network is an important concept in the study of brain mechanisms underlying disrupted anatomical and functional brain connectivity in many neurological diseases [13, 14]. It describes the human brain as a large, interacting, and complex network characterized by highly coordinated, efficient, and integrated neuronal activities among specialized and widely distributed cerebral cortices [15]. The fcMRI is used to characterize the synchrony and intercorrelation of these brain networks.

Dysfunction of neuronal networks had been found to be associated with clinical symptoms such as fatigue and depression, and could therefore provide potential treatment monitoring and evaluation [16, 17]. Many previous work and neurobiological reviews in chapter 1 implied that functional networks of DMN, hypothalamus, thalamus and hippocampus might be damaged following the neurodegenerative injuries and could lead to the clinical symptoms in mild traumatic brain injury (MTBI), post-traumatic stress disorder (PTSD) [18], mild cognitive impairment (MCI) and multiple sclerosis (MS) [18-23]. The purpose of the present study was to identify the resting networks connecting from these four regions (i.e., DMN, hypothalamus, thalamus and hippocampus), and detect the network connectivity abnormalities using advanced quantitative MRI techniques-fcMRI in the four representative neurodegenerative diseases. Additionally, voxel-wise fractional amplitude of low frequency fluctuation (fALFF) method was also implemented to examine any local regional activity injuries [24].

METHODS

Participants

For MTBI data, twenty-seven patients (mean age of 33.4 ± SD 11.2 years; 6 female and 21 males) and 27 demographically similar healthy controls (mean age of 35.4 ± SD 11.4 years; 13 female and 14 males) were involved in this study. The institutional review board approved this study, and written informed consent forms of all study subjects were obtained after the nature of this study was explained to the subjects before participation. Inclusion criteria are as follows: closed head injury with either posttraumatic amnesia of less than 24 hours or loss of consciousness of approximately 30 minutes or less, with a Glasgow Coma Scale (GCS) score between 13 and 15. Exclusion criteria included a history of alcohol or drug abuse; a preexisting psychiatric disorder; a prior brain injury other than the current episode; and a history of other neurologic disease, including stroke, epilepsy, and somatic disorders.

The mean interval between MRI and trauma for MTBI patients in this study was 23 days (range: 3–58 days); and the mean loss of consciousness duration was 12 min (range: 1–30 min). All patients were recruited from a level I trauma center and sustained MTBI defined by clinical criteria [1] with GCS score between 13 and 15, and had various posttraumatic symptoms. The injury mechanisms of patients included 8 motor vehicle accidents, 7 assaults, 6 falls, 3 sports related, 2 bicycle collisions, 1 other, and the location of injury included 3 on the left side, 9 on the right side, 5 on the back, 2 on the forehead, 8 of other regions of the brain. Neuropsychological tests were performed within 24 hour of the MRI scan for each subject including six types of neuropsychological tests and post concussion syndrome (PCS) clinical measure. Posttraumatic symptoms including anxiety, depression, and fatigue were assessed using self-report questionnaires and scales, for which higher scores indicate greater symptomatology. MTBI patients showed significantly increased PCS scores compared with controls ($P = 0.003$) [17, 24].

For PTSD data, participants were identified using the clinician-administered PTSD scale (CAPS) within DSM-IV criteria (e.g., CAPS score > 40) [25]. RS-fMRI data of 52 controls (age: 70.0 ± SD 4.8 years; 51 men and 1 women) and 18 PTSD patients (age: 68.6 ± SD 4.1 years; 18 men) were analyzed. Patients had significantly higher CAPS score than controls (75.4 ± 4.9 in PTSD vs. 29.9 ± 4.7 in controls, P = 0.00004). In addition to imaging, all participants completed several neuropsychological questionnaires, including Everyday Cognition (ECog), Clinical Dementia Rating (CDR), Mini-Mental State Examination (MMSE), Montreal Cognitive Assessment (MOCA), Alzheimer's Disease Assessment Scale–Cognitive (ADAS-Cog), Geriatric Depression Scale (GDS), Functional Assessment Questionnaire (FAQ), Combat Exposure Scale (CES), and the Armed Forces Qualification Test (AFQT) [25]. All participants were also assessed using a battery of neuropsychological tests including the clock drawing test, the Rey auditory verbal learning test, the category fluency test, the trail making test and the Boston naming test. All PTSD data were obtained from the ADNI-DOD which is a multi-modal (MRI, PET and neuropsychological assessment), nonrandomized study that recruited War veterans selected from the Department of Veterans Affairs compensation and pension records, investigating TBI and/or PTSD as potential risk factors for the development of AD. ADNI-DOD is part of the ADNI project [22, 26].

For the MCI data, thirteen early AD patients (age: 76.2 ± SD 8.4 years, Mini-Mental State Examination [MMSE] score < 24), 17 patients with MCI (age: 76.7 ± SD 5.5 years, MMSE: 24–28), and 14 age-matched healthy controls (age: 76.3 ± SD 8.25 years, MMSE > 28) from the Alzheimer's Disease neuroimaging initiative (ADNI) database (http://ida.loni.usc.edu) were used in this study [27]. Data were selected based on age ranges of subjects as well as availability of four imaging modalities for the same subject during the period of October 2010 to August 2013. MR/PET Imaging ADNI Data used in the preparation of this article were obtained from the ADNI database (http://www.adni.loni.ucla.edu). The primary goal of ADNI has been to test whether serial MRI, positron emission tomography (PET), other biological markers, and clinical and neuropsychological assessment can be combined to measure the progression of mild cognitive impairment (MCI) and early Alzheimer's disease (AD).

Part of the data for PTSD and MCI/AD project used in preparation of this chapter were obtained from the ADNI database with permission. ADNI is the result of efforts of many co-investigators from a broad range of academic institutions and private corporations, and subjects have been recruited from over 50 sites across the United States and Canada. For up-to- date information, see http://ida.loni.usc.edu or www.adni-info.org.

For the MS data, twenty-four patients with clinically definite relapsing-remitting MS (mean age, 38.25 ± SD 9.23 years; 18 women and 6 men) and 24 age-matched healthy volunteers (mean age, 38.46 ± SD 10.52 years; 10 women and 14 men) were recruited. None of the patients with MS had any evidence of prior diagnosis of cardiovascular morbidity, cerebrovascular disease, or other neurologic diseases. All patients displayed a characteristic phenotype that included but was not limited to visual disturbances (e.g., diplopia), paresthesias, ataxia, dysphagia, fatigue, and nonspecific disabling arthralgias. The patients had a varied degree of previous symptoms with an average Expanded Disability Status Scale (EDSS) score of 2.47 (range, 0–6). The average disease duration for the patient group was 5.12 years (range, 0.67–14 years). The institutional review board approved this study. All participants gave informed consent after the nature of the procedure had been fully explained [28].

Imaging Acquisition

All MRI experiments were performed in the 3T MRI scanner. MR images were acquired using a body coil for transmission and a 12-element SENSE coil for reception. For MTBI and MS data of RS-fMRI, a standard gradient-echo EPI (TR/TE = 2000/30 ms, number of volumes = 153, flip angle = 75°, FOV = 220 x 220 mm^2, matrix = 128 x 128, 153 volumes) was performed in axial plane parallel to a line passing through the anterior-posterior commissure (AC-PC line) with 5 mm slice thickness and 1mm gap and positioned to cover nearly the entire cerebrum, resulting in a spatial resolution of 1.72 x1.72 x 6 mm^3 and acquisition time of 5 minutes and 6 seconds. All patients and healthy subjects were instructed to close their eyes but stay awake during the resting-state fMRI imaging examination. The 3D Magnetization-prepared rapid acquisition gradient-echo (MPRAGE) (TR/TE/TI = 2300/2.98/900 ms, flip angle = 9°, resolution = 1x1x1mm^3) was used as reference image for overlaying RS-fMRI connectivity maps and also for the anatomical normalization of seed-based fcMRI. Conventional imaging, including T2-weighted fast spin-echo and fluid-attenuated inversion recovery images (FLAIR, TR/TE/TI = 9200/82/2500 ms; flip angle = 150°; resolution = 0.86 x 0.86 x 3 mm^3), was also obtained for lesion load quantification. Susceptibility-weighted imaging sequences (SWI, 1st echo TE = 4.92 ms, 6th echo TE = 46.74 ms, echo spacing = 6.97 ms, TR = 51ms; flip angle = 15°; resolution = 0.5 x 0.5 x 2.0 mm^3; 52 axial sections) were also implemented with high spatial resolution to help detect hemorrhagic or other lesions.

For the PTSD and MCI data, RS-fMRI (TR/TE = 3000/30 ms, flip angle1 = 80°, 3.3 mm isotropic spatial resolution with 48 slices and 140 volumes), T1-MPRAGE (acquired sagittally using volumetric 3D sequence with 0.94 x 0.94 mm^2 in-plane spatial resolution, 1.2 mm slice thickness with matrix size of 256 x 256 and 166 slices), and T2-weighted axial FLAIR images (TR/TE = 9000/90ms, flip angle = 90°, 0.86 x 0.86 mm^2 in-plane spatial resolution, 5 mm thick and 35 slices) were obtained with 3T MRI units at multiple ADNI centers with standardized imaging protocols across sites and platforms.

Image Post-Processing and Data Analysis

Four fcMRI networks were derived for further data processing. For the DMN fcMRI and seed mask image derivation, two regions of interest, including the MPFC seed (MNI: 0, 48, 23 mm) and the PCC seed (MNI: 26, 248, 39 mm), both with 896-mm^3 volumes, were derived from the script seed library and were well evaluated previously by Fox and Raichle [10]. Since the individual seeding approach with the seed placed within either the PCC or the MPFC generates different and incomplete DMN connectivity patterns, the combined seed (Figure 1a) from two core MPFC and PCC seeds was used to generate a comprehensive DMN pattern [17].

This combined DMN template had been used for single-participant independent component analysis (ICA) automatic template matching and component selection, and could further validate the seed-based DMN pattern recognition. The ICA method can help separate the whole-brain signal fluctuations from physiologic noise and automatically capture the entire DMN as a single major component using the comprehensive template generated from the combined seed [17, 27].

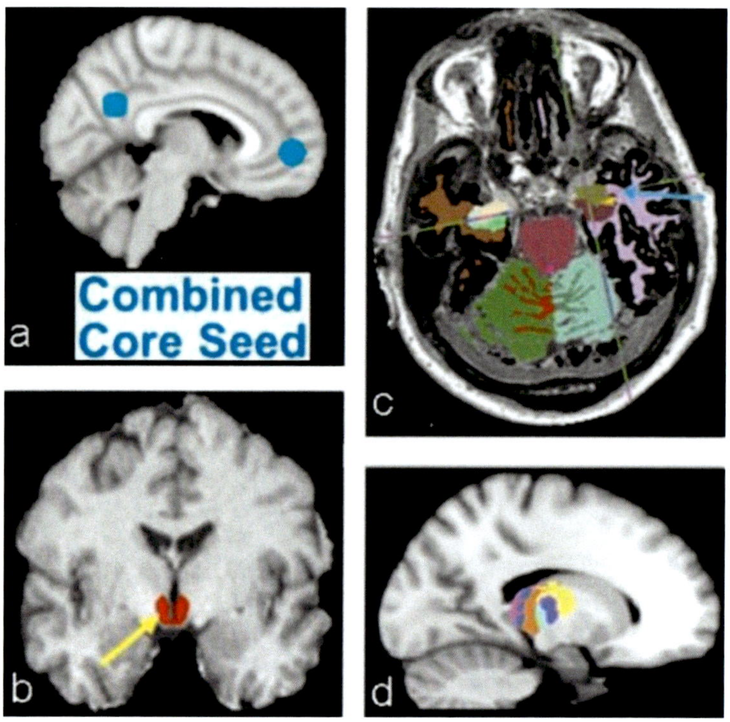

Figure 1. Four seed images for fcMRI computation: a. Default mode network (DMN) seed combining the medial prefrontal and posterior cingulate core seeds; b. Hypothalamus (red region of interest); c. Hippocampus (arrows); and d. Thalamus (seven colored sub-segments).

Hypothalamus mask was obtained with in-house developed probability mask that were averaged from 81 young normal control participants with the 75% probability map (Figure 1b). Briefly, for each of the 81 subjects, hypothalamus was first manually delineated with the MEDx software (http://medx.sensor.com) based on the MPRAGE image in the coronal view at individual space after intensity inhomogeneity correction. The anatomical MPRAGE image was then normalized to the Montreal Neurological Institute (MNI) 2-mm template space, and the same transformation was applied to the individual hypothalamic mask. Group average of the hypothalamic maps was obtained in the MNI template space, and 75% probabilistic threshold was applied to derive the hypothalamic ROI in the template space as shown in Figure 1b.

Two other conventional seeds including the hippocampal formation (HF, Figure 1c) from the script seed library (http://www.nitrc.org/projects/fcon_1000), and the thalamus from the FSL (www.fmrib.ox.ac.uk/fsl) template based on diffusion data were derived for fcMRI computation (Figure 1d). DMN was the conventionally task-negative network, while the other three seeds including hypothalamus, hippocampal formation and thalamus generated task-positive fcMRI networks that were more active at task conditions in contrast to the resting state.

The RS-fMRI data were preprocessed with motion correction and outlier screening such as mean frame displacement (FD) < 0.6 mm to remove excessive motion [17]. We used 3D high resolution T1-MPRAGE for image coregistration and normalization. To generate fcMRI map using seed-based analysis, Pearson's correlation between the preprocessed average time series of the pre-selected seed as in Figure 1 and each voxel within the whole brain area was computed. The resultant values of Z-transformed (using Fisher's r-to-z transform) map were used for subsequent group-level post-hoc statistical analysis. Some relatively new methods including ICA and graph-theory based small-worldness network analysis were performed as well for further functional and systematic investigation [13, 17, 29]. ICA is a more robust technique involving the blind source separation method that captures the essential components of multivariate resting-state functional MR imaging data. To validate our findings, we used three different strategies of ICA, template-based ICA method, hybrid ICA seed-based method, and group ICA method, in patients with MTBI compared with healthy individuals, using the automatic detection algorithm for component selection [17].

In addition to fcMRI, the factional amplitude of low frequency fluctuation (fALFF) was calculated from RS-fMRI to reflect the intensity of regional spontaneous brain activity or neuronal activation. The idea of the fALFF method was to scale the summary of amplitude at the low-frequency band (e.g., 0.01–0.08 Hz) to the summary of amplitude across the whole frequency of the time course of each voxel to remove white and physiological noise [24].

RESULTS

1. Resting-State fcMRI Patterns of Four Seeds and fALFF in Controls

Significant statistical comparison results were derived with $T > 2.35$, $P < 0.01$; with red color representing regions of positive connectivity from the seed and blue color representing regions of negative connectivity.

DMN pattern seeding from the core seed demonstrated positive connectivity with the MPFC, PCC, inferior parietal lobe, temporal cortex including hippocampus and orbitofrontal cortex, but negative with DAN, front eye field (FEF), visual cortex and cerebellum (Figure 2).

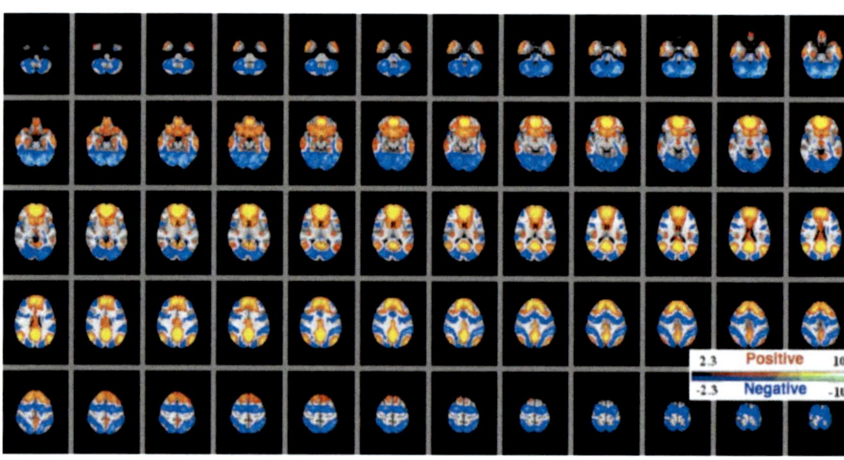

Figure 2. DMN fcMRI group mean pattern of controls (P<0.01).

Regarding the hypothalamic RSN connectivity pattern, positive connectivity with the peri-hypothalamic regions including thalamus, hippocampus, orbitofrontal cortex, and small areas in the medial prefrontal and posterior cingulate cortices, but negative with visual cortex and superior parietal lobe were observed (Figure 3).

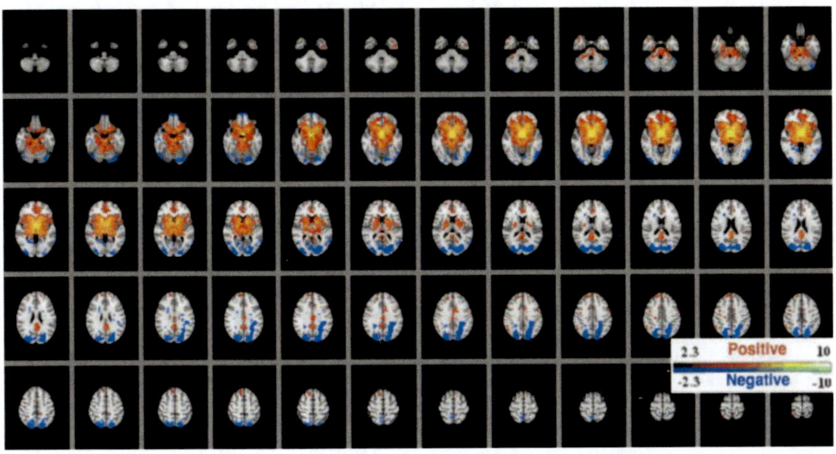

Figure 3. Hypothalamic fcMRI group mean pattern of controls (P<0.01).

Hippocampal RSN connectivity pattern includes positive connectivity with the temporal cortex and posterior cingulate, but negative connectivity with DAN, central executive network and visual cortex (Figure 4).

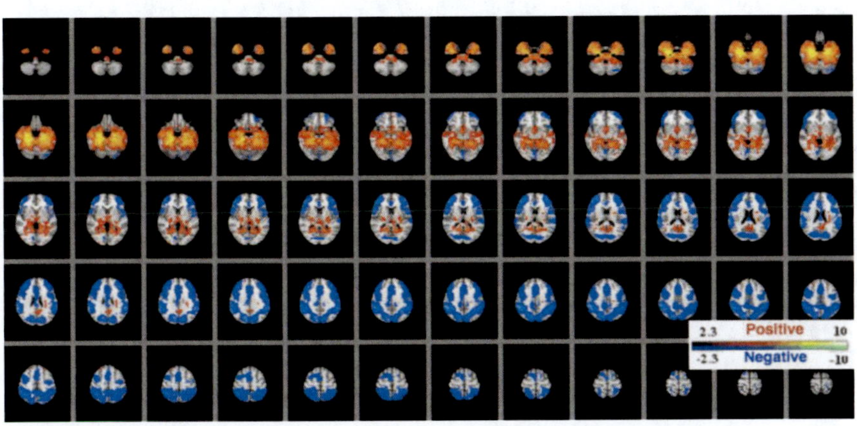

Figure 4. Hippocampal fcMRI group mean pattern of controls (P<0.01).

For the thalamic RSN, positive connectivity with the peri-thalamic regions, cerebellum, inferior temporal cortex and posterior cingulate, but negative connectivity with central executive network, frontal and visual cortices were found (Figure 5).

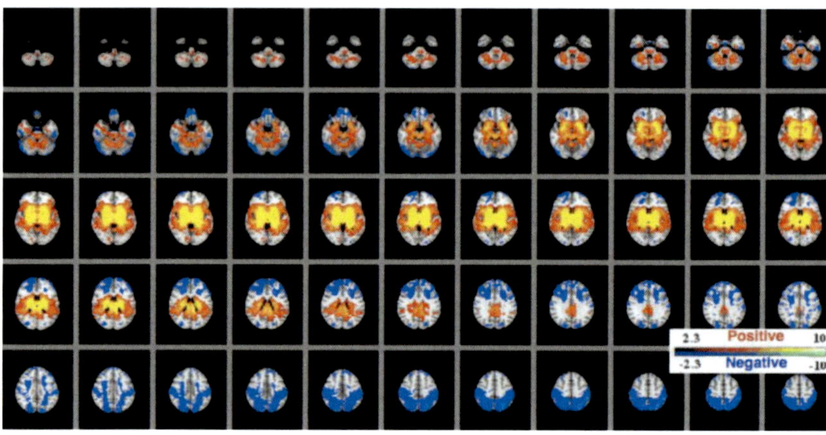

Figure 5. Thalamic fcMRI group mean pattern of controls (P<0.01).

Based on fALFF, pattern of positive and higher spontaneous neuronal activity in the thalamus and cortical gray matter including occipital, parietal and superior frontal regions, but lower and negative in the inferior temporal cortex, cerebellar and orbitofrontal regions was found (Figure 6).

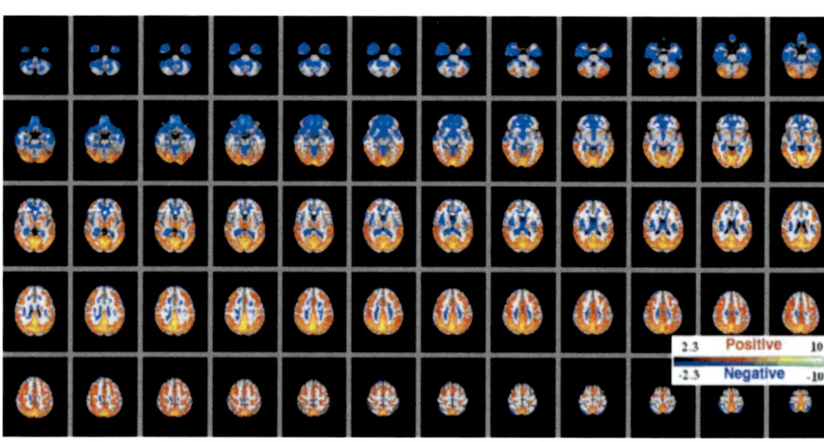

Figure 6. fALFF group mean pattern of controls (P<0.01).

2. fcMRI and fALFF differences between PTSD Patients and Controls

Significant statistical comparison results were derived with T > 2.35, P < 0.01; with red color representing regions of lower fcMRI strength in patients compared to controls and blue color representing regions of higher fcMRI strength in patients compared to controls.

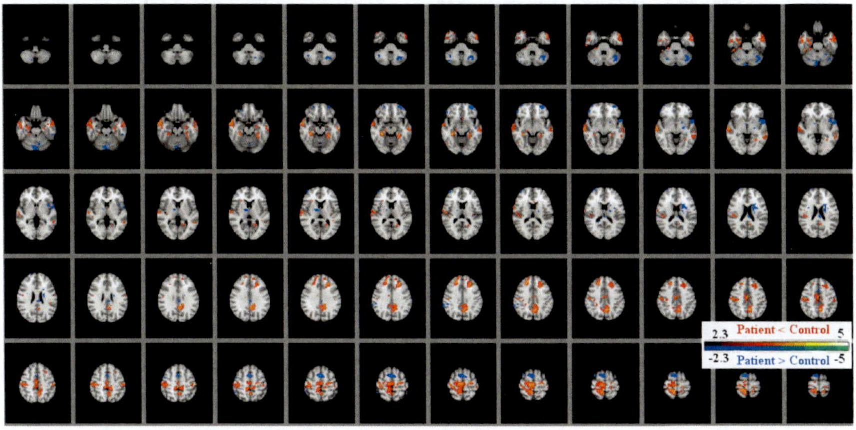

Figure 7. DMN differences comparing PTSD patients to controls ($P < 0.01$).

Compared to healthy controls, PTSD patients showed decreased DMN connectivity, especially in the posterior cingulate, medial prefrontal and temporal cortices, motor and supplementary motor areas (Figure 7; red color, $P < 0.01$). In contrast, there were also increased DMN connectivity in the vmPFC, cerebellum and small regions in the thalamus and superior frontal cortex in PTSD patients (Figure 7; blue color).

In PTSD patients, hypothalamic fcMRI was reduced in the small temporal regions, midbrain including pons, cerebral peduncle and substantia nigra, small superior frontal and right Broca's areas, bilateral motor and supplementary motor areas, but increased in the vmPFC, hippocampus, small peri-ventricular regions, and occipital cortex (Figure 8; $P < 0.01$).

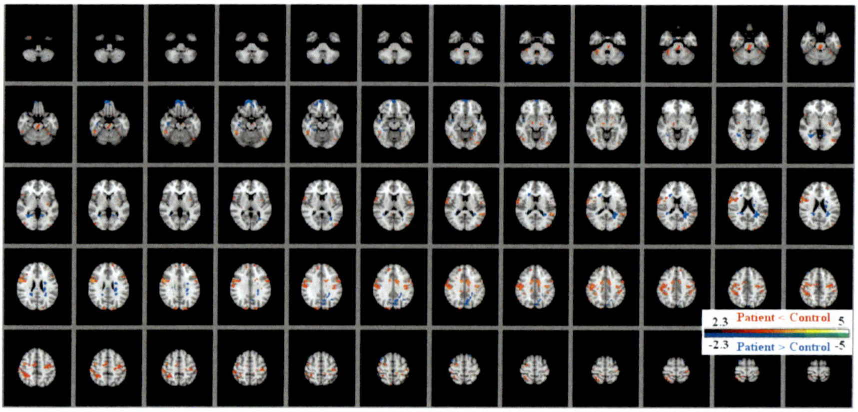

Figure 8. Hypothalamic fcMRI differences comparing PTSD patients to controls (P < 0.01).

PTSD patients also showed decreased hippocampal fcMRI in the vmPFC and temporal cortex, but increased fcMRI in the bilateral parietal and cerebellar regions (Figure 9). And finally thalamic fcMRI showed decreased connectivity in the temporal, subcortical caudate and putamen, somatosensory and premotor (middle cingulate) cortices in PTSD patients in comparison to controls, but increased fcMRI in the vmPFC, cerebellum and inferior orbito-prefrontal regions (Figure 10).

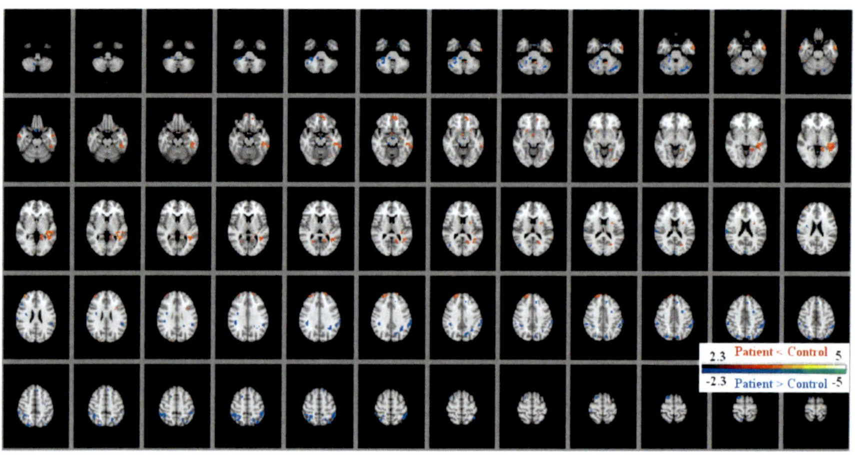

Figure 9. Hippocampal fcMRI differences comparing PTSD patients to controls (P < 0.01).

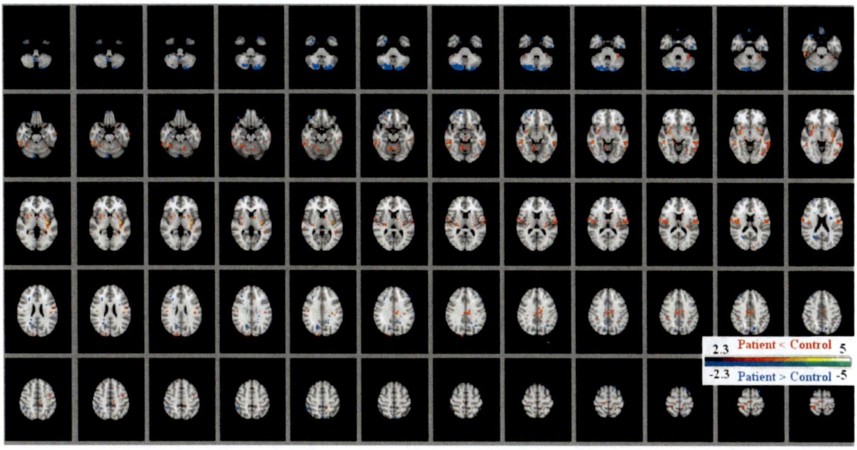

Figure 10. Thalamic fcMRI differences in PTSD patients compared to controls ($P < 0.01$).

Based on fALFF, PTSD patients showed decreased functional activity (i.e., neuronal activation) in the medial prefrontal cortex, superior portion of vmPFC, amygdala, hippocampus, and superior temporal regions, but increased functional activity in small regions in the gyrus rectus, inferior parietal, angular and occipital regions compared to controls (Figure 11; $P < 0.01$).

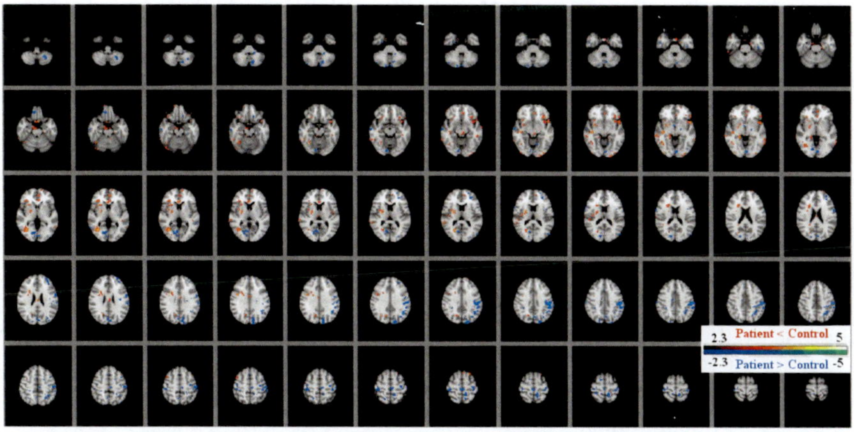

Figure 11. fALFF differences in PTSD patients compared to controls.

3. fcMRI and fALFF Differences between MTBI Patients and Controls

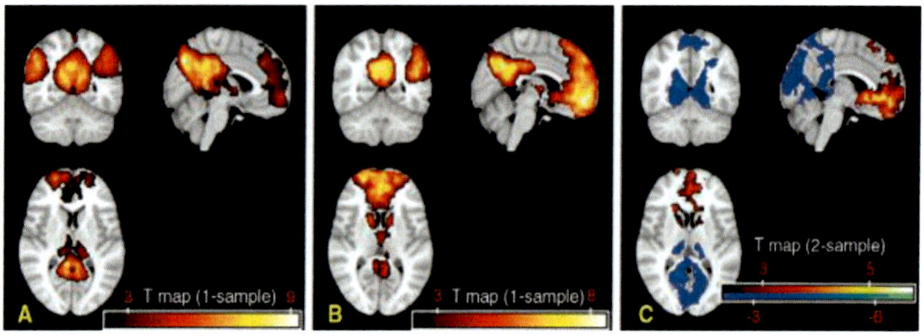

Figure 12. DMN templates obtained with the hybrid ICA seed method in patients and control subjects (corrected, $P < 0.05$; $K \geq 20$). A, Typical but enhanced connectivity pattern of the DMN was identified in the healthy control group. B, Disrupted DMN pattern is shown in the patient group. C, Group-level voxel-wise image of hybrid DMN template differences comparing MTBI to control groups. Red = increased functional connectivity, blue = decreased functional connectivity in patients compared with control subjects. These changes in DMN pattern were consistent with the single-subject ICA results by means of visual inspection [17, 30].

When compared with the control subjects, there was significantly reduced connectivity in the PCC and parietal regions but increased frontal connectivity around the MPFC in patients with MTBI ($P < 0.01$; **Figure** 12), using hybrid seed-based ICA method. Three different algorithms of ICA including single-participant subject ICA, hybrid seed-based ICA and group ICA had been tested to covalidate the fcMRI findings. And all results were consistent and independent of data processing algorithms, which suggested posterior hypoconnectivity and anterior hyperconnectivity in MTBI [17]. Furthermore, these fronto-posterior opposing changes within the DMN were significantly correlated ($r = -0.44$, $P = 0.03$). There was a significant correlation after Bonferroni correction between decreased DMN in the posterior regions with the Trail Making Test B (Pearson correlation coefficient, $r = 0.60$; corrected $P = 0.02$), which is a measure of executive functioning to assess mental flexibility - specifically, the ability to shift rapidly between cognitive sets. By using covariance analysis, a significant correlation ($P < 0.01$) between functional connectivity MR imaging (z score) of anterior MPFC and clinical symptoms, including anxiety, depression, fatigue, and post-concussive symptoms, was also observed. For instance, a negative correlation between MPFC connectivity and depression score in patients was found with MTBI (Spearman correlation coefficient, r = -0.56; corrected, P = 0.01), indicating that patients with higher MPFC functional connectivity had a lower degree of depression.

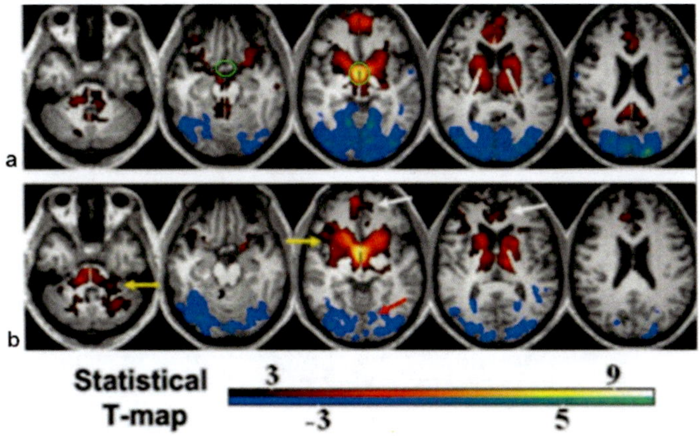

Figure 13. Hypothalamic fcMRI in controls (a) and MTBI patients (b) using seed-based one-sample t-test and corrected $P < 0.05$. Green circle in (a) marks the hypothalamic ROI. Red-yellow color indicates positive correlation, while blue-cyan indicates negative correlation. There was significantly decreased connectivity in MTBI in both positive (white arrows) and negative (red arrow) networks and increased RSN (yellow arrows) using a two-sample t-test ($P < 0.05$). [Source Image: reference [29]; use with permission]

Using seed-based methods, a symmetric normal pattern of hypothalamic connectivity of both positive and negative correlations was shown in healthy control group (corrected $P < 0.05$, $K > 20$; Figure 13a) [29]. The functional network with positive correlation primarily involved brain stem, deep gray matter, and several focal cortical areas. More specifically, these regions include bilateral hypothalamus, tuberomamillary nucleus, thalamus, putamen, caudate, basal forebrain, medial prefrontal and inferior parietal cortex, small superior amygdala region; the locus coeruleus in the medial portion of brain stem, and raphe nuclei. The functional network with negative correlation primarily involved the visual and primary motor cortices. Compared to control group, MTBI group (corrected $P < 0.05$, $K > 20$; Figure 13b) showed disrupted hypothalamic fcMRI, which demonstrated significantly decreased positive connectivity in the medial prefrontal cortex, inferior posterior parietal and cingulate regions but increased connectivity in the peri-hypothalamic regions and cerebellum. In addition, the patient group also showed significantly decreased negative RSNs in the visual and bilateral premotor areas (corrected $P < 0.05$).

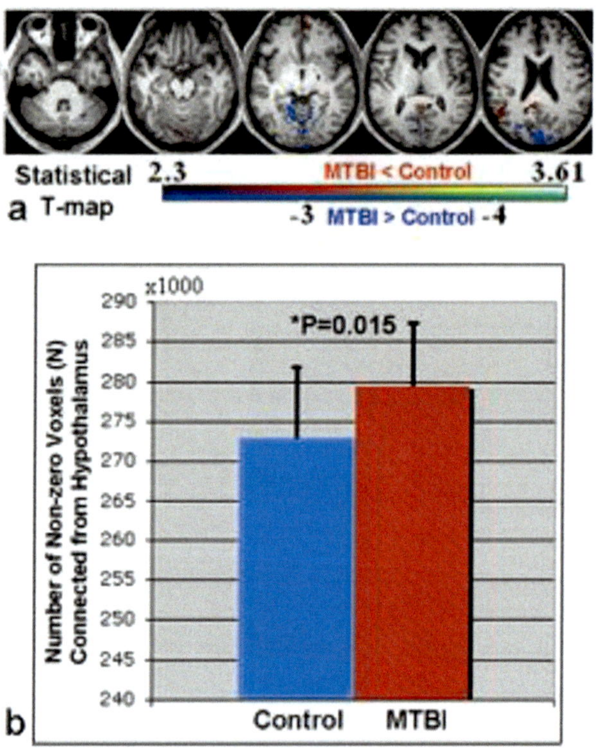

Figure 14. a: Statistical difference map comparing hypothalamic fcMRI between two groups (red-yellow indicates CT > MTBI contrast while blue-cyan indicates CT < MTBI with cluster corrected $P < 0.05$). b: Globally, the number of voxels connected from hypothalamus to the whole brain with nonzero correlation was also significantly higher in MTBI patients compared to controls ($P = 0.015$). [Source Image: reference [29]; use with permission]

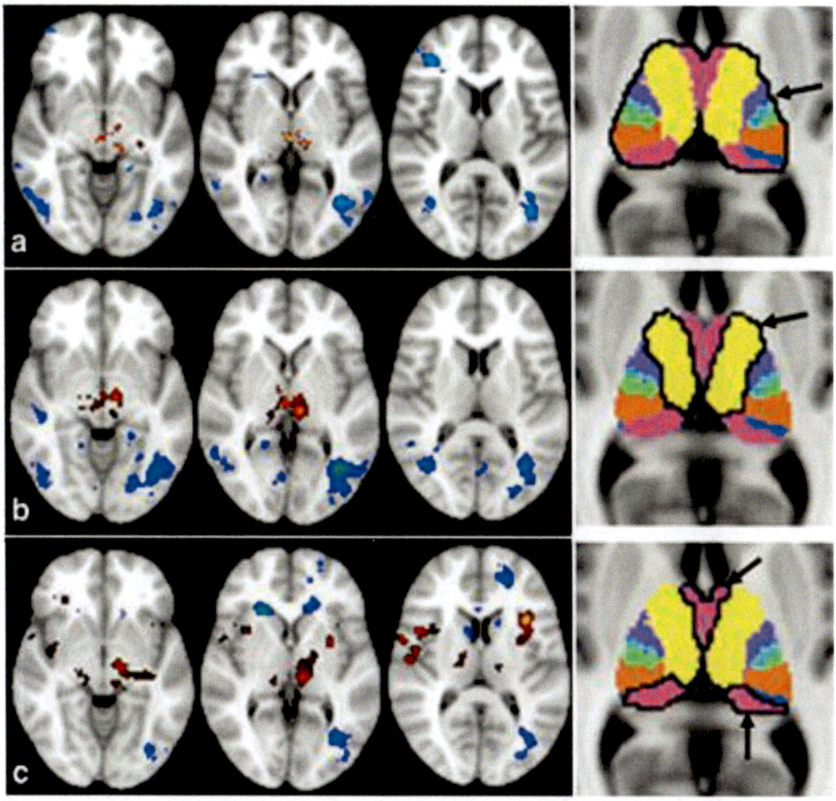

Figure 15. Based on RS-fMRI, selected slices covering thalamic regions compared fcMRI of MTBI and controls; seeding from bilateral thalamus and its segments (i.e., 4 and 7) marked with a black margin on the rightmost images. a: RS-fcMRI seeding from the whole thalamus showed differences between MTBI patients and controls; with decreased thalamo-thalamo connectivity (red color) and mainly increased thalamo-occipital connectivity (blue color) in MTBI patients compared with controls (minimum $Z > 2.3$; cluster significance, $P < 0.05$, corrected; cluster size $K > 100$) with a 25% gray matter mask from the FSL standard template. b: Thalamic segment 4 fcMRI when seed was put in the sub-segment 4 (frontal projections) showed more reduced thalamo-thalamo connectivity in red color comparing patients to controls; and similar increased thalamo-occipital connectivity in blue color. C: RS-fcMRI when seed was put in the sub-segment 7 (temporal projections) showed thalamic fcMRI differences between MTBI patients and controls with decreased thalamo-thalamo connectivity (red color), while more increased thalamo-cortical connectivity (occipital and scattered frontal white matter regions) in MTBI patients compared with controls. [Source Image: reference [24]; use with permission]

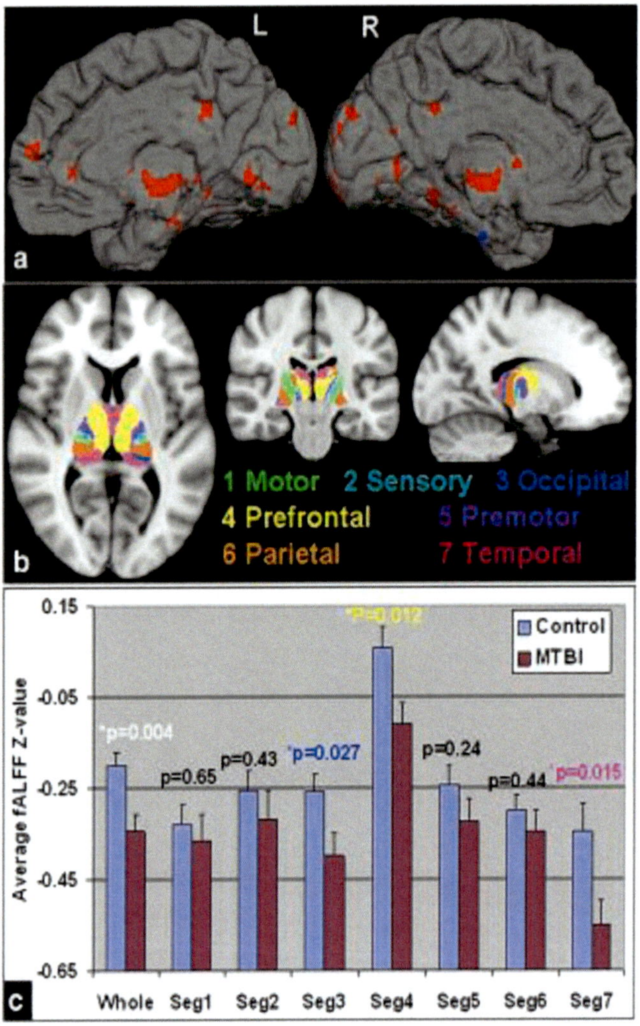

Figure 16. a: An fALFF analysis based on RS-fMRI comparing MTBI with controls in the whole brain showed mostly reduced fALFFs in the thalamus, medial frontal, occipital, and temporal regions (red color) (minimum Z > 2.3; cluster significance, P < 0.05, corrected). Shown are the medial surface projection views on the left and right hemispheres; and in the seven specific thalamic segments according to the FSL template. (b) There were significantly reduced fALFFs in the overall thalamus and its segments for occipital (template index number 3), frontal [4], and temporal [7] projections in MTBI patients compared with controls (P < 0.05). (c) As the fALFFs were z-standardized over the whole brain; the negative values indicated that the thalamic fALFFs were less than the whole brain average. [Source Image: reference [24]; use with permission]

Figure 14a shows the statistical difference image comparing the functional connectivity maps seeded from hypothalamus between the two groups with control > MTBI shown in warm red color that mainly localizes in temporal, medial prefrontal, posterior cingulate, right inferior parietal, supplementary motor, and control < MTBI shown in blue color primarily in the visual and bilateral premotor areas (corrected $P < 0.05$, $K > 20$, 25% gray matter mask) [29]. There was significantly higher number of hypothalamic-connected voxels (i.e., fcMRI) in MTBI patients compared to control group (279282 ± 7990 vs. 272813 ± 9012, $P = 0.015$) (Figure 14b), which might come from the reduced suppression of occipital cortex connections in MTBI as shown in Figure 14b. In patients with MTBI, there was a significantly higher fatigue z-score than the control group (28.0 ± 16.2 vs. 16.0 ± 8.0, $P = 0.005$).

No significant differences of hippocampal fcMRI between MTBI patients and controls were found ($P > 0.05$). Regarding thalamic fcMRI, there was significantly reduced thalamo-thalamo fcMRI seeding from the thalamus (Figure 15a) in the MTBI patients compared with controls, as well as seeding from its segments for frontal (segment 4) (Figure 15b) and temporal (FSL segment 7) (Figure 15c) projections compared with controls (corrected $P < 0.05$) based on RS-fMRI [17, 24]. There was also decreased thalamo-cortical fcMRI in the frontal and temporal regions in the MTBI patients; with increases of fcMRI in the occipital and parietal regions (including scattered frontal white matter regions).

Based on RS-fMRI data, whole brain voxel-based analysis showed that MTBI patients demonstrated significantly decreased fALFF in regions including thalamus, scattered regions in medial frontal, temporal, and occipital cortices (Figure 16a) compared with controls (minimum $Z > 2.3$; cluster significance, $P < 0.05$, corrccted). More specifically, there was a significant reduction in fALFF in the entire bilateral thalamus ($P = 0.004$) (Figure 16b), as well as in thalamic segments projecting to frontal (FSL thalamic template index 4) ($P = 0.012$), temporal (FSL thalamic template index 7) ($P = 0.015$), and occipital cortices (FSL thalamic template index 3) ($P = 0.027$), in MTBI patients compared with controls (Figure 16c). At finger-tapping task condition, a significant increase in fALFFs in the thalamus, motor, and supplementary motor areas during finger-tapping compared with resting state (one-sample paired t-test; $P < 0.05$, $K > 20$) in the control subjects. In MTBI patients, the fALFF difference map between finger-tapping and resting state RS-fMRI showed less fALFF change in the thalamus (almost no activity) and primary motor areas as well as less de-activation of default mode network areas when compared with controls ($P < 0.05$, $K > 20$) [17, 24].

4. fcMRI and fALFF Differences between MCI Patients and Controls

Significant statistical comparison results were derived with $T > 2.35$, $P < 0.01$; with red color representing regions of lower fcMRI strength in patients compared to controls and blue color representing regions of higher fcMRI strength in patients compared to controls.

Compared to controls, MCI patients showed decreased fcMRI in the bilateral hippocampus, medial prefrontal cortex and posterior cingulate ($P < 0.01$, Figure 17; red). MCI patients also had increased fcMRI in the inferior temporal, orbitofrontal cortex, dorsolateral prefrontal cortex and superior parietal regions (Figure 17; blue).

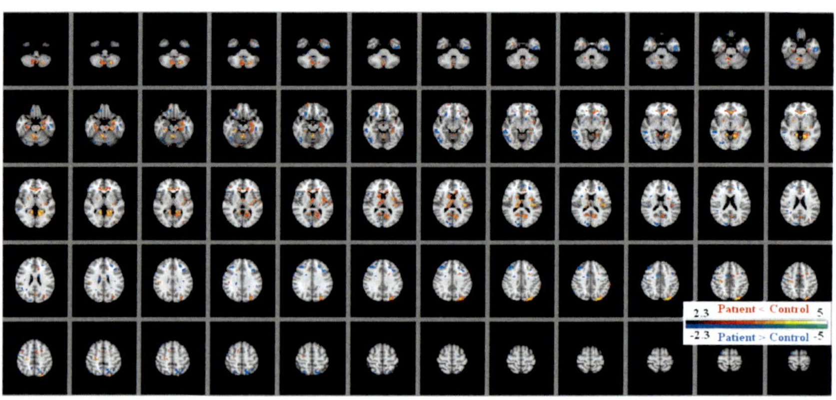

Figure 17. DMN differences comparing MCI to controls ($P < 0.01$).

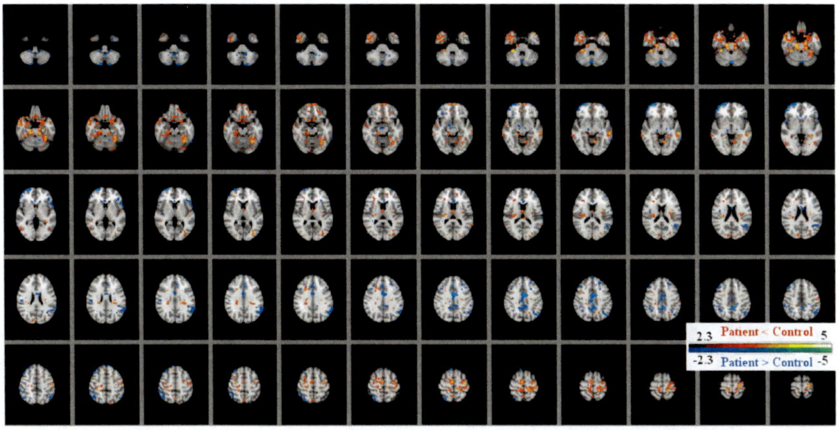

Figure 18. Hypothalamic fcMRI differences in MCI patients vs. controls ($P < 0.01$).

Comparing MCI to controls, patients had decreased hypothalamic fcMRI in large temporal regions including amygdala and hippocampus, vmPFC, medial prefrontal cortex, bilateral inferior parietal cortex and supplementary motor area, but slightly increased fcMRI in the dorsolateral prefrontal, cingulate, cuneus, cerebellum, and superior parietal regions (Figure 18).

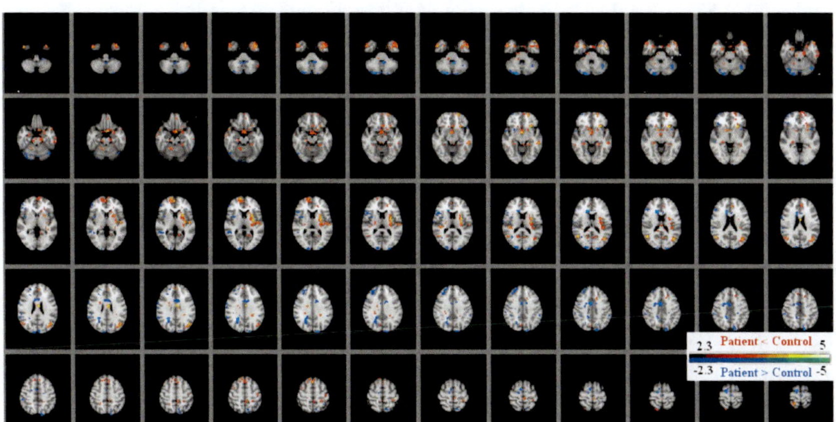

Figure 19. Hippocampal fcMRI differences comparing MCI vs. controls ($P < 0.01$).

Comparing MCI vs. controls, patients had decreased hippocampal fcMRI in the temporal cortex including hippocampus, hypothalamus and medial prefrontal cortex. Increased fcMRI in the cerebellum, dorsolateral prefrontal, superior parietal and supplementary motor regions had been observed as well (Figure 19; $P < 0.01$).

MCI patients showed reduced thalamic fcMRI in the regions of inferior temporal cortex, posterior cingulate and midbrain, but increased thalamic fcMRI in the bilateral dorsolateral prefrontal and parietal cortices (Figure 20).

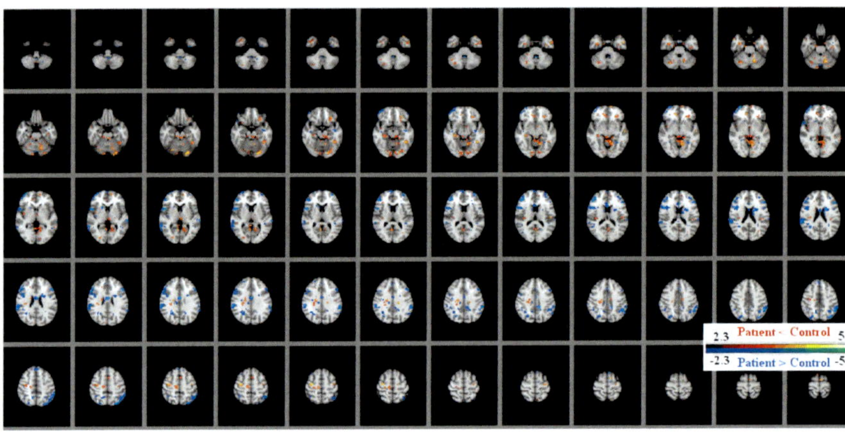

Figure 20. Thalamic fcMRI differences in MCI patients compared to controls ($P < 0.01$).

As of fALFF, MCI patients had reduced functional activity in the regions of medial prefrontal, temporal cortex including hippocampus and superior segment and parietal cortex, but increased functional activity in the regions of inferior temporal cortex and paracentral motor areas (Figure 21; $P < 0.01$) in comparison to controls.

In addition, a significant correlation was found between white matter lesion load (WMLL) and DMN connectivity strength ($r = 0.56$; $P = 0.02$), as well as between WMLL and fALFF activity values ($r = 0.63$; $P = 0.01$) in MCI patients [27]. Meanwhile, in AD patients, a marginal interregional correlation exists between the RS-fMRI fALFF activity value averaged over the reduced and increased regions ($r = -0.46$; $P = 0.11$). A significant correlation was found between amyloid load of the whole cerebral cortex and mean fALFF activity value from the lower difference regions in AD patients (r = 0.64; P = 0.046).

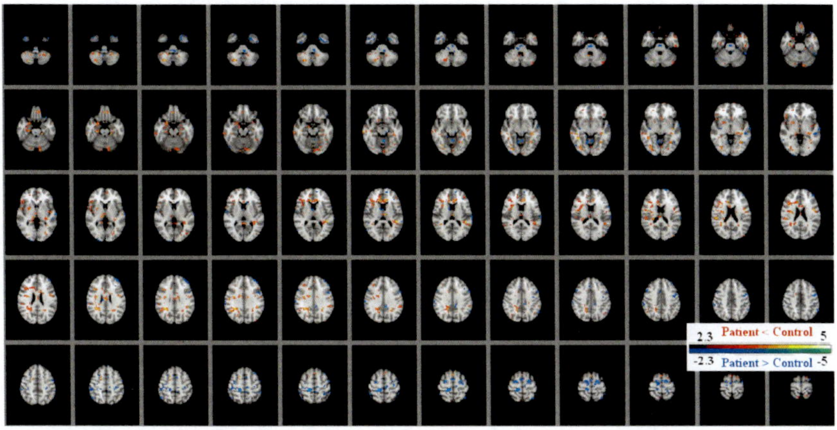

Figure 21. fALFF differences in MCI patients compared to controls (P < 0.01).

5. fcMRI and fALFF Differences between MS Patients and Controls

Significant statistical comparison results were derived with T > 2.35, P < 0.01; with red color representing regions of lower fcMRI strength in patients compared to controls and blue color representing regions of higher fcMRI strength in patients compared to controls.

Compared to age-matched controls, MS patients presented decreased DMN fcMRI in the medial prefrontal, middle cingulate and supplementary motor area, but increased DMN in the cerebellum and small regions in inferior temporal and occipital cortices (Figure 22; P < 0.01).

Comparing to controls, MS patients had slightly decreased hypothalamic fcMRI in the midbrain, inferior temporal and supplementary motor areas and cerebellum, but increased fcMRI in the midbrain and small regions in striatum and motor areas (Figure 23; P < 0.01).

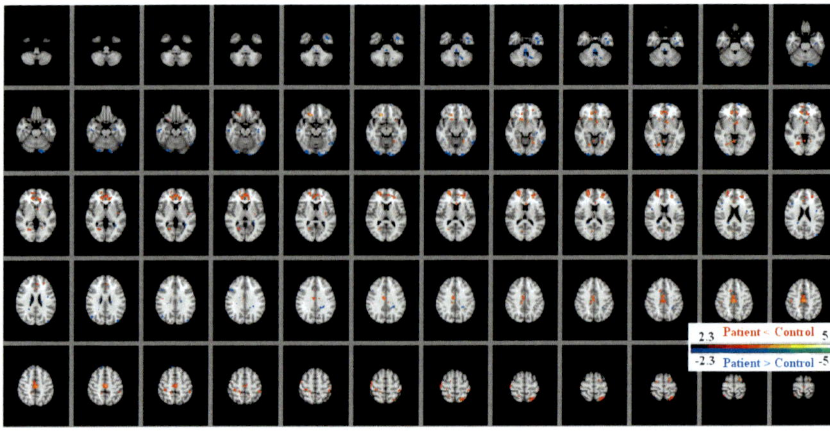

Figure 22. DMN differences comparing MS to controls (T > 2.35, P < 0.01).

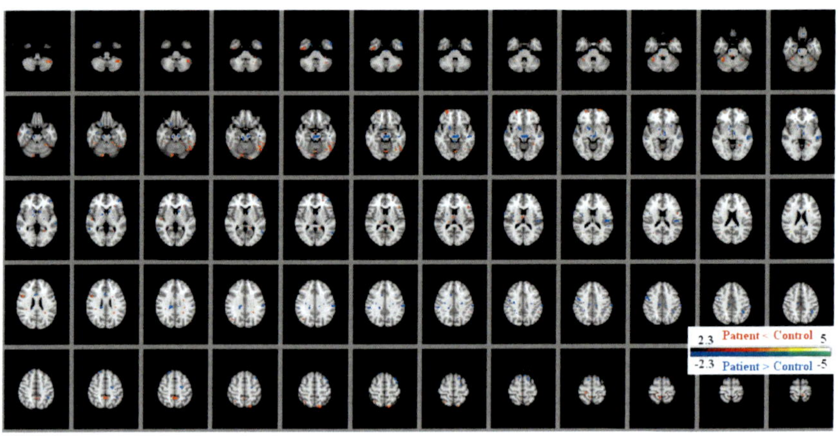

Figure 23. Hypothalamic fcMRI differences in MS patients vs. controls (P < 0.01).

MS patients showed decreased hippocampal fcMRI in the occipital, superior parietal and post-central regions, but increased fcMRI in the DMN regions and cerebellum compared to controls (Figure 24).

Comparing MS patients to control group, thalamic connectivity network showed decreased fcMRI in vmPFC, small regions in medial prefrontal cortex, insula, ventral striatum (VST), Broca's area, superior temporal and occipital regions; but increased fcMRI in the cerebellum, dorsolateral prefrontal cortex, superior parietal and precuneus regions (Figure 25).

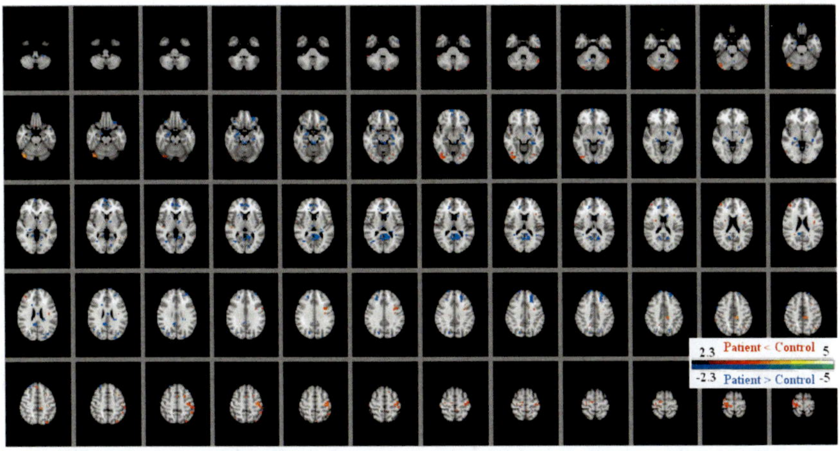

Figure 24. Hippocampal fcMRI differences comparing MS to controls (P < 0.01).

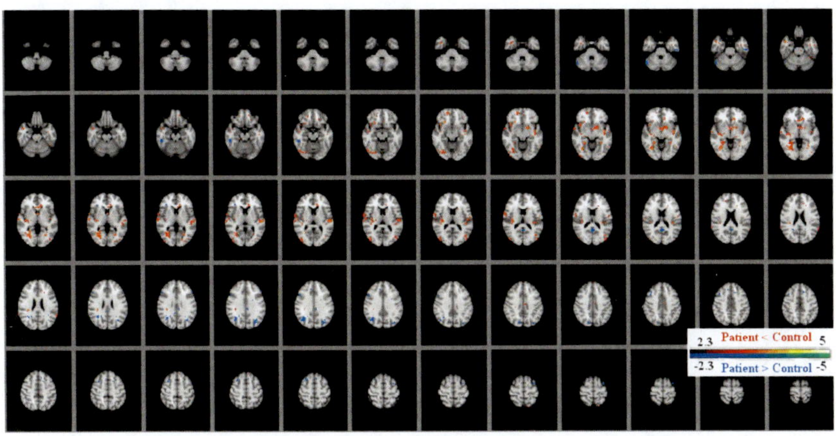

Figure 25. Thalamic fcMRI differences in MS patients compared to controls (P <0.01).

Finally, based on fALFF, MS patients showed decreased functional activity in the small regions in the somatosensory cortex, superior parietal lobe, occipital cortex and temporal-occipital junction and cerebellum, but increased functional activity in small regions in the inferior orbitofrontal including vmPFC, temporal, medial prefrontal regions and striatum compared to controls (Figure 26; P < 0.01).

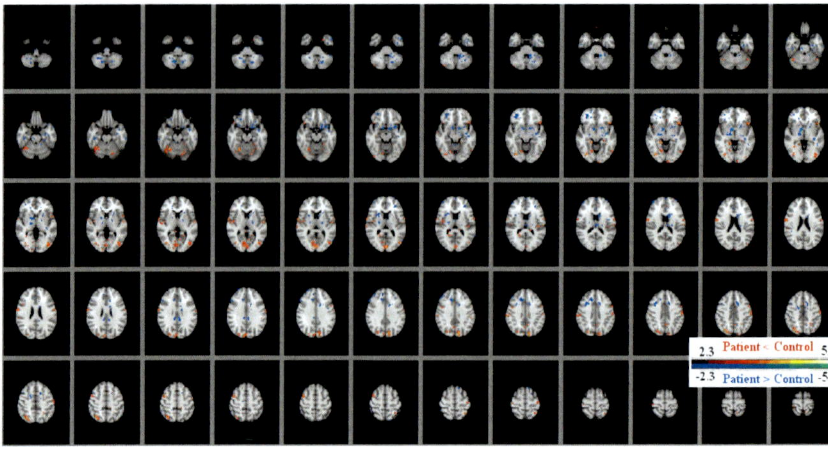

Figure 26. fALFF differences in MS patients compared to controls ($P < 0.01$).

DISCUSSION

In MTBI patients, DMN fcMRI showed significant negative correlation between increased MPFC functional connectivity and decreased PCC functional connectivity in comparison to controls, and suggested that fronto-posterior DMN nodes are not only intrinsically interdependent but also highly complementary in their functions. Increased MPFC activation has been reported previously in moderate and severe traumatic brain injury [31], and is hypothesized to represent brain neuroplasticity operating in recovery and neural repair after injury [1, 32]. In addition, the reduced posterior connectivity correlated positively with neurocognitive dysfunction (e.g., cognitive flexibility), while the increased frontal connectivity correlated negatively with post-traumatic symptoms (i.e., depression, anxiety, fatigue, and post-concussion syndrome). Our finding of a negative correlation between increased MPFC connectivity and neuropsychologic symptoms also supports the notion of increased usage of MPFC neural resources as compensation in response to the impaired neurocognitive function [17]. Previous studies, outside of traumatic brain injury, have also shown MPFC connectivity changes in patients with anxiety and depression, although the pattern of changes in connectivity appears to be different compared with MTBI [5, 33, 34]. The abnormally increased MPFC usage over the long run, however, might lead to persistent psychologic symptoms, such as the depression, anxiety, and fatigue seen in these patients.

The changes of hypothalamic RSNs in patients suggest disrupted intrinsic functional networks after brain injury, consistent with recent findings [24, 35]. The significantly decreased functional connectivity with basal forebrain (one of the orexin projecting sites) and medial prefrontal area in MTBI may be due to direct injury (i.e., diffuse axonal injury), while decreased negative connectivity in occipital regions in MTBI is probably due to the reduced anti-phase synchronization between hypothalamus and occipital cortex [24]. However, increased hypothalamic connectivity within peri-hypothalamic regions and cerebellum and global fcMRI from hypothalamic may indicate the compensative mechanism with functional reorganization or hypothalamic reactivity after injury. Direct localization of the hypothalamus with fMRI experiment such as visual food demonstrated lower hypothalamic activity in MTBI patients compared to controls [14]. Our recent results also demonstrated both microstructural and functional connectivity abnormalities of hypothalamus in these MTBI patients with relatively early stage after injury (<2 months), indicating RS-fMRI have the potential to provide objective connectivity measures in patients with hypothalamic symptoms which are difficult to explain with conventional MR imaging [29]. Injury to the hypothalamus can occur following a traumatic accident through either shearing that cause diffuse axonal injury within its pathway and damage to its cell bodies which extends through the skull due to the coup/contre-coup forces [36, 37]. In the case of MTBI, it is now believed that even when no evidence based on conventional methods including imaging of hypothalamic dysfunction, repeated screening should be conducted up to 3 years post-injury in order to detect the development of hypothalamic symptoms due to the potential subclinical damage causing apoptosis and atrophy in the hypothalamus [38]. On the other hand, as expected, there was no significant dysfunction of hippocampal fcMRI in the MTBI patient population, suggesting the memory cognitive function was maintained as confirmed by the no significant memory dysfunction in these patients at the initial visits [10].

The decreased thalamo-frontal and thalamo-temporal fcMRI, and fALFF reduction covalidates that these areas may be more predisposed to injury [39]. It is known that the frontal and temporal lobes are at increased risk of contusion in moderate and severe injury; and hypometabolism in the thalamus and frontal and temporal lobes had also been reported in severe TBI patients based on PET FDG uptake imaging [39-43]. Our results of abnormal fALFFs and fcMRI indicate that the thalamo-cortical network is disrupted in patients shortly after MTBI both in strength and in spatial extent and these changes may be related to the neuropsychological origins of PCS in these patients. Along with abnormal thalamic activation during task, the current study also showed significantly reduced fALFFs in the thalamus, predominantly in segments 3, 4, and 7, in MTBI patients as compared with healthy controls. Correspondingly, we also found disrupted thalamo-cortical connectivity and reduced thalamo-thalamo fcMRI in patients with the most abnormal patterns within segments 4 and 7. Segments 4 and 7 represent the medial frontal and medial dorsal subdivisions of the thalamus, which relay inputs from the amygdala and project to the prefrontal cortex and the limbic system. As a result, these nuclei in particular play a crucial role in attention, planning, organization, abstract thinking, and active memory, domains in which patients with MTBI often have deficits. The reduced thalamic fALFFs in patients corroborate with previous notion that the thalamus is injured after MTBI and, furthermore, reduced fALFFs suggest that this thalamic injury may be the primary cause of significantly disrupted thalamo-cortical functional connectivity as observed in this study and a previous study [34].

Although PTSD and TBI are highly prevalent comorbid conditions in especially combat-related military veterans and have some overlapping neuropsychiatric symptoms such as dementia and distress [20, 21, 44], the neuroimaging manifestation of each type is distinguishable with different neuronal network utilization and rerouting. For the PTSD patients, we found reliable DMN fcMRI reduction in the core regions including both PCC and MPFC, with fcMRI increment in the anti-correlated inferior orbitofrontal, thalamus, and supplementary motor cortices, compared to controls. Higher hypothalamic functional connectivities with the vmPFC, midbrain and occipital cortex connectivities were observed in PTSD patients as well. On the other hand, lower fcMRI between hypothalamus, somatosensory cortex, Broca's area, and bilateral motor/supplementary motor areas were found in patients compared to controls. These fcMRI deficits suggested there might be motor and auditory processing deficits in PTSD patients. PTSD patients also showed decreased hippocampal fcMRIs with vmPFC and temporal somatosensory/motor cortices, but increased hippocampal fcMRI with the bilateral parietal and cerebellar regions. Lower thalamic fcMRI in the temporal and middle cingulate cortices in PTSD patients, but higher thalamic fcMRI in the cerebellum and small orbitofrontal regions were observed, consistent with the hypoconnectivity from the thalamus observed [16]. Furthermore, based on fALFF results, PTSD patients had less functional activities (i.e., neuronal activation) in the medial prefrontal cortex including vmPFC, amygdala, hippocampus, and superior temporal regions, but more activities in the cerebellum, inferior parietal, angular and occipital regions. Consistent with previous studies [22, 26, 45-47], dysfunction of multiple neuronal networks including DMN, hippocampus, vmPFC and amygdala regions in PTSD patients was illustrated. Especially decreased DMN and hypothalamic fcMRIs, but increased hippocampal and vmPFC connectivity as well as compensated cerebellar and parietal/occipital activations had been observed [19, 48]. Both lower vmPFC and hippocampal connectivities and activities suggested possible local neuronal injury in addition to the pathway damage occurred in these regions affecting memory and emotion regulation functions, as well as post-traumatic depression, anxiety and fatigue symptoms.

MCI patients had decreased hippocampal fcMRI in the temporal cortex including hippocampus, hypothalamus and medial prefrontal cortex, but increased fcMRI in the cerebellum, superior frontal and parietal, as well as supplementary motor regions. The hippocampal fcMRI results in this study are in agreement with previous studies indicating that reductions in conductivity from both the PCC and hippocampus to the whole brain as well as between these two regions might be primary factors in episodic memory impairment associated with early AD [9]. It had recently been reported that high correlation between the PCC and the hippocampus with delayed free recall supported the assumption that these two regions of the brain might play an important role in episodic memory, encoding and retrieval, comprehension and production of narrative speech, and speech perception [29, 33]. Moreover, the PCC and hippocampus are commonly shown to be active in tasks involving cognitive control, verbal and working memory, as well as visual processing [49, 50], which might further the use of this methodology in diagnostic and classification procedures. Our findings were in-line with the literature, suggesting possible functional rerouting, compensatory and neuroplasticity mechanism in response to the accumulation of amyloid plaques and tau tangles in early AD [25, 51-53].

Compared to controls, MCI patients also showed significantly lower DMN fcMRI in the bilateral hippocampus, medial prefrontal cortex and posterior cingulate, with higher connectivity in the inferior temporal, orbitofrontal and superior parietal regions. And MCI patients had significantly lower hypothalamic fcMRI in the temporal cortex including hippocampus as well, and other cerebellum and supplementary motor area, accompanied with higher fcMRI in the inferior frontal, cingulum and parietal regions [24]. Furthermore, MCI patients showed reduced thalamic fcMRI in the regions of inferior temporal cortex and midbrain, but increased thalamic fcMRI in the bilateral superior frontal and parietal cortices. Furthermore, based on fALFF, MCI patients had reduced functional activity in the regions of medial prefrontal, temporal cortex including hippocampus and superior temporal regions, but increased functional activity in the regions of inferior temporal cortex and paracentral motor areas. Consistent with previous findings, the DMN RS-fMRI results showed reduced functional connectivity in the MPFC region and reduced functional activity by means of fALFF in the temporal region in MCI patients compared with controls [49, 54]. The fALFF was also reduced in the temporal region in AD compared with MCI patients, but increased in the parietal region [27]. Deficits in the key regions that play important roles in memory, motivation and executive function including hippocampus, medial prefrontal cortex, hypothalamus and posterior cingulate in MCI patients are expected where MCI and AD patients often demonstrate atrophy and degeneration [55]. Our results also complement the previous findings with high detection sensitivities and confirmative results such as lower fcMRI between hippocampus and hypothalamus (both ways with similar results found seeding from either region), as well as lower activity in the temporal cortex at early stage of dementia [56-58]. The typical brain networks dysfunction including DMN regions such as posterior cingulate and medial prefrontal cortex, as well as largely involved temporal cortex including hippocampal fcMRI, especially hypoconnectivities and lower activities among these regions, imply that these four neuronal networks can be used to detect brain abnormality in MCI efficiently with high sensitivity.

Compared to age-matched controls, MS patients presented decreased DMN fcMRI in the medial prefrontal and cingulum, but increased fcMRI in the cerebellum and small regions in inferior temporal and occipital cortices. MS patients also had slightly decreased hypothalamic fcMRI in the cerebellum, inferior temporal and supplementary motor areas, but increased fcMRI in the midbrain and small regions in striatum and motor areas. Furthermore, decreased hippocampal fcMRI in the occipital, superior parietal and post-central regions, but increased hippocampal fcMRI in the DMN and cerebellum were found in patients. And finally, comparing MS patients to control group, thalamic connectivity showed decreased fcMRI in distributed regions in orbitofrontal, striatum, superior temporal, and occipital regions; but increased fcMRI in the cerebellum, dorsolateral prefrontal cortex, superior parietal and precuneus regions. MS patients also showed decreased fALFF functional activity in the somatosensory cortex, superior parietal and occipital cortices as well as temporal-occipital junction, but increased functional activity in small regions in the vmPFC, inferior orbitofrontal, temporal, frontal regions and striatum ($P < 0.01$). Impairments of connectivity and activity in the occipital, motor and temporal regions, especially neuronal networks identified from the four selected seeds, were consistent with the clinical symptoms of MS patients such as visual and motor disabilities [59-63].

CONCLUSION

The fcMRI results support the concept that functional networks of DMN, thalamic, hypothalamic and hippocampal connectivity, frontal and temporal cortical functional activity are involved in injury after MTBI or PTSD at variable degrees. And these imaging biomarkers may play a crucial role in elucidating the pathomechanisms of post concussion syndrome, dementia or stress disorder in these patients. Our results of disruption of functional and structural hypothalamic connectivity and activity in patients with MTBI as well as significant correlations with post-concussion syndrome might help to resolve an array of clinical symptoms in MTBI related to sleep disturbance and fatigue. In PTSD patients, various abnormal functional activity and connectivities had been observed, including decreased DMN and hippocampal fcMRI but increased hypothalamic and vmPFC connectivity, together with compensated cerebellar and occipital activations, but lower vmPFC, hippocampal and amygdala activities. MCI patients also had significantly lower fcMRI from the hippocampus and key memory regions such as medial prefrontal cortex, hypothalamus and posterior cingulate. Our data also provided preliminary evidence of the potential usefulness of fcMRI analyses for the detection of abnormalities of functional coordination in MS. It had been demonstrated that the fcMRI patterns including DMN and thalamic connectivity as well as regional functional activity were altered in patients with MS, especially in the occipital and motor regions. Such observations can increase the understanding of structural and functional deficits in MS. All the results in this study were consistent with previous findings, with some distinctive neuronal network differences found in each type of disease. Specific regional connectivity and activity patterns of neuronal networks and comprehensive applications will help to distinguish and diagnose more accurately each type of the four neurodegenerative diseases with various etiologies including traumatic accident, stress disorder, dementia and inflammation.

ACKNOWLEDGMENTS

Data collection and sharing for this project was funded by the Alzheimer's Disease Neuroimaging Initiative (ADNI) (National Institutes of Health Grant U01 AG024904) and DOD ADNI (Department of Defense award number W81XWH-12-2-0012). ADNI is funded by the National Institute on Aging, the National Institute of Biomedical Imaging and Bioengineering, and through generous contributions from the following: AbbVie, Alzheimer's Association; Alzheimer's Drug Discovery Foundation; Araclon Biotech; BioClinica, Inc.; Biogen; Bristol-Myers Squibb Company; CereSpir, Inc.; Cogstate; Eisai Inc.; Elan Pharmaceuticals, Inc.; Eli Lilly and Company; EuroImmun; F. Hoffmann-La Roche Ltd and its affiliated company Genentech, Inc.; Fujirebio; GE Healthcare; IXICO Ltd.; Janssen Alzheimer Immunotherapy Research and Development, LLC.; Johnson and Johnson Pharmaceutical Research and Development LLC.; Lumosity; Lundbeck; Merck and Co., Inc.; Meso Scale Diagnostics, LLC.; NeuroRx Research; Neurotrack Technologies; Novartis Pharmaceuticals Corporation; Pfizer Inc.; Piramal Imaging; Servier; Takeda Pharmaceutical Company; and Transition Therapeutics. The Canadian Institutes of Health Research is providing funds to support ADNI clinical sites in Canada. Private sector contributions are facilitated by the Foundation for the National Institutes of Health (www.fnih.org). The grantee organization is the Northern California Institute for Research and Education, and the study is coordinated by the Alzheimer's Therapeutic Research Institute at the University of Southern California. ADNI data are disseminated by the Laboratory for NeuroImaging at the University of Southern California.

Data used in preparation of this article were obtained from the Alzheimer's Disease Neuroimaging Initiative (ADNI) database website (adni.loni.usc.edu). The author is one of the investigators of ADNI data cohort. The other investigators within the ADNI might contribute to the design and implementation of ADNI and/or provide data but did not participate in analysis or writing of this report.

REFERENCES

[1] Raichle ME, Snyder AZ. A default mode of brain function: a brief history of an evolving idea. *Neuroimage* 2007;37:1083-1090; discussion 1097-1089.

[2] Damoiseaux JS, Rombouts SA, Barkhof F, et al. Consistent resting-state networks across healthy subjects. *Proc Natl Acad Sci U S A* 2006;103:13848-13853.

[3] Cordes D, Haughton VM, Arfanakis K, et al. Frequencies contributing to functional connectivity in the cerebral cortex in "resting-state" data. *AJNR Am J Neuroradiol* 2001;22:1326-1333.

[4] Biswal B, Yetkin FZ, Haughton VM, Hyde JS. Functional connectivity in the motor cortex of resting human brain using echo-planar MRI. *Magn Reson Med* 1995;34:537-541.

[5] Greicius MD, Flores BH, Menon V, et al. Resting-state functional connectivity in major depression: abnormally increased contributions from subgenual cingulate cortex and thalamus. *Biol Psychiatry* 2007;62:429-437.

[6] de Lecea L, Kilduff TS, Peyron C, et al. The hypocretins: hypothalamus-specific peptides with neuroexcitatory activity. *Proc Natl Acad Sci U S A* 1998;95:322-327.

[7] Zhou J, Jaquet A, Bissagnene E, et al. Short-term risk of anaemia following initiation of combination antiretroviral treatment in HIV-infected patients in countries in sub-Saharan Africa, Asia-Pacific, and central and South America. *J Int AIDS Soc* 2012;15:5.

[8] Mantini D, Perrucci MG, Del Gratta C, Romani GL, Corbetta M. Electrophysiological signatures of resting state networks in the human brain. *Proc Natl Acad Sci U S A* 2007;104:13170-13175.

[9] Zhou Y, Dougherty JH, Jr., Hubner KF, Bai B, Cannon RL, Hutson RK. Abnormal connectivity in the posterior cingulate and hippocampus in early Alzheimer's disease and mild cognitive impairment. Alzheimers Dement 2008;4:265-270.

[10] Fox MD, Raichle ME. Spontaneous fluctuations in brain activity observed with functional magnetic resonance imaging. *Nature Reviews Neuroscience* 2007;8:700-711.

[11] Greicius MD, Krasnow B, Reiss AL, Menon V. Functional connectivity in the resting brain: a network analysis of the default mode hypothesis. *Proc Natl Acad Sci U S A* 2003;100:253-258.

[12] Raichle ME, MacLeod AM, Snyder AZ, Powers WJ, Gusnard DA, Shulman GL. A default mode of brain function. *Proc Natl Acad Sci U S A* 2001;98:676-682.

[13] Zhou Y, Lui YW. Small-World Properties in Mild Cognitive Impairment and Early Alzheimer's Disease: A Cortical Thickness MRI Study. *ISRN Geriatr* 2013; 542080.

[14] Zhou Y. *Neuroimaging in Multiple Sclerosis.* Nova Science Publishers 2017.

[15] Adamantidis A, de Lecea L. The hypocretins as sensors for metabolism and arousal. *J Physiol* 2009;587:33-40.

[16] Lanius RA, Frewen PA, Tursich M, Jetly R, McKinnon MC. Restoring large-scale brain networks in PTSD and related disorders: a proposal for neuroscientifically-informed treatment interventions. *Eur J Psychotraumatol* 2015;6:27313.

[17] Zhou Y, Milham MP, Lui YW, et al. Default-mode network disruption in mild traumatic brain injury. *Radiology* 2012;265:882-892.

[18] Dean KR, Hammamieh R, Mellon SH, et al. Multi-omic biomarker identification and validation for diagnosing warzone-related post-traumatic stress disorder. *Mol Psychiatry* 2019.

[19] Rowland JA, Stapleton-Kotloski JR, Alberto GE, et al. Contrasting Effects of Posttraumatic Stress Disorder and Mild Traumatic Brain Injury on the Whole-Brain Resting-State Network: A Magnetoencephalography Study. *Brain Connect* 2017;7:45-57.

[20] Schneider ALC, Ling G. Associations of TBI, PTSD, and depression with dementia risk among female military veterans: Not just men. *Neurology* 2019;92:117-118.

[21] Qureshi KL, Upthegrove R, Toman E, Sawlani V, Davies DJ, Belli A. Post-traumatic stress disorder in UK civilians with traumatic brain injury: an observational study of TBI clinic attendees to estimate PTSD prevalence and its relationship with radiological markers of brain injury severity. *BMJ Open* 2019;9:e021675.

[22] Weiner MW, Harvey D, Hayes J, et al. Effects of traumatic brain injury and posttraumatic stress disorder on development of Alzheimer's disease in Vietnam Veterans using the Alzheimer's Disease Neuroimaging Initiative: Preliminary Report. *Alzheimers Dement* (N Y) 2017;3:177-188.

[23] Filippi M, Bruck W, Chard D, et al. Association between pathological and MRI findings in multiple sclerosis. *Lancet Neurol* 2019;18:198-210.

[24] Zhou Y, Lui YW, Zuo XN, et al. Characterization of thalamo-cortical association using amplitude and connectivity of functional MRI in mild traumatic brain injury. *J Magn Reson Imaging* 2014;39:1558-1568.

[25] Mohamed AZ, Cumming P, Gotz J, Nasrallah F, Department of Defense Alzheimer's Disease Neuroimaging I. Tauopathy in veterans with long-term posttraumatic stress disorder and traumatic brain injury. *Eur J Nucl Med Mol Imaging* 2019;46:1139-1151..

[26] Weiner MW, Veitch DP, Hayes J, et al. Effects of traumatic brain injury and posttraumatic stress disorder on Alzheimer's disease in veterans, using the Alzheimer's Disease Neuroimaging Initiative. *Alzheimers Dement* 2014;10:S226-235.

[27] Zhou Y, Yu F, Duong TQ, Alzheimer's Disease Neuroimaging I. White matter lesion load is associated with resting state functional MRI activity and amyloid PET but not FDG in mild cognitive impairment and early Alzheimer's disease patients. *J Magn Reson Imaging* 2015;41:102-109.

[28] Zhou Y, Milham M, Zuo XN, et al. Functional Homotopic Changes in Multiple Sclerosis with Resting-State Functional MR Imaging. *AJNR Am J Neuroradiol* 2013.

[29] Zhou Y. Abnormal structural and functional hypothalamic connectivity in mild traumatic brain injury. *J Magn Reson Imaging* 2017;45:1105-1112.

[30] Zhou Y. *Neuroimaging in Mild Traumatic Brain Injury.* Nova Science Publishers 2017.

[31] Christodoulou C, DeLuca J, Ricker JH, et al. Functional magnetic resonance imaging of working memory impairment after traumatic brain injury. *J Neurol Neurosurg Psychiatry* 2001;71:161-168.

[32] Scheibel RS, Newsome MR, Steinberg JL, et al. Altered brain activation during cognitive control in patients with moderate to severe traumatic brain injury. *Neurorehabil Neural Repair* 2007;21:36-45.

[33] Broyd SJ, Demanuele C, Debener S, Helps SK, James CJ, Sonuga-Barke EJ. Default-mode brain dysfunction in mental disorders: a systematic review. *Neurosci Biobehav Rev* 2009;33:279-296.

[34] Zhao XH, Wang PJ, Li CB, et al. Altered default mode network activity in patient with anxiety disorders: an fMRI study. *Eur J Radiol* 2007;63:373-378.

[35] Hahnel S, Herweh C. MRI biomarkers in mild traumatic brain injury. *Neurology* 2015;84:554-555.

[36] Kolassa IT, Wienbruch C, Neuner F, et al. Altered oscillatory brain dynamics after repeated traumatic stress. *BMC Psychiatry* 2007;7:56.

[37] Yount R, Raschke KA, Biru M, et al. Traumatic brain injury and atrophy of the cingulate gyrus. *J Neuropsychiatry Clin Neurosci* 2002;14:416-423.

[38] Long JA, Watts LT, Chemello J, Huang S, Shen Q, Duong TQ. Multiparametric and longitudinal MRI characterization of mild traumatic brain injury in rats. *J Neurotrauma* 2015;32:598-607.

[39] Silver JM, McAllister TW, Yudofsky SC. *Textbook of Traumatic Brain Injury.* American Psychiatric Publishing, Inc. 2011;2nd Edition.

[40] Crochet S, Fuentealba P, Cisse Y, Timofeev I, Steriade M. Synaptic plasticity in local cortical network in vivo and its modulation by the level of neuronal activity. *Cereb Cortex* 2006;16:618-631.

[41] Garcia-Panach J, Lull N, Lull JJ, et al. A voxe-based analysis of FDG-PET in traumatic brain injury: regional metabolism and relationship between the thalamus and cortical areas. *Journal of Neurotrauma* 2011;28:1707-1717.

[42] Haacke EM, Duhaime AC, Gean AD, et al. Common data elements in radiologic imaging of traumatic brain injury. *J Magn Reson Imaging* 2010;32:516-543.

[43] Schiff ND. Bringing neuroimaging tools closer to diagnostic use in the severely injured brain. *Brain* 2007;130:2482-2483.

[44] Merritt VC, Jurick SM, Crocker LD, et al. Evaluation of objective and subjective clinical outcomes in combat veterans with and without mild TBI and PTSD: A four-group design. *J Clin Exp Neuropsychol* 2019;41:665-679.

[45] Zuj DV, Felmingham KL, Palmer MA, et al. Neural activity and emotional processing following military deployment: Effects of mild traumatic brain injury and posttraumatic stress disorder. *Brain Cogn* 2017;118:19-26.

[46] Mohamed AZ, Cumming P, Gotz J, Nasrallah F, Department of Defense Alzheimer's Disease Neuroimaging I. Tauopathy in veterans with long-term posttraumatic stress disorder and traumatic brain injury. *Eur J Nucl Med Mol Imaging* 2019;46:1139-1151.

[47] Negreira AM, Abdallah CG. A Review of fMRI Affective Processing Paradigms Used in the Neurobiological Study of Posttraumatic Stress Disorder. *Chronic Stress (Thousand Oaks)* 2019;3.

[48] Young KD, Zotev V, Phillips R, Misaki M, Drevets WC, Bodurka J. Amygdala real-time functional magnetic resonance imaging neurofeedback for major depressive disorder: A review. *Psychiatry Clin Neurosci* 2018;72:466-481.

[49] Buckner RL, Snyder AZ, Shannon BJ, et al. Molecular, structural, and functional characterization of Alzheimer's disease: evidence for a relationship between default activity, amyloid, and memory. *J Neurosci* 2005;25:7709-7717.

[50] Mosconi L, Berti V, Glodzik L, Pupi A, De Santi S, de Leon MJ. Pre-Clinical Detection of Alzheimer's Disease Using FDG-PET, with or without Amyloid Imaging. *Journal of Alzheimer's Disease* 2010;20:843-854.

[51] Jack CR, Jr., Knopman DS, Jagust WJ, et al. Hypothetical model of dynamic biomarkers of the Alzheimer's pathological cascade. *Lancet Neurol* 2010;9:119-128.

[52] Villemagne VL, Okamura N. Tau imaging in the study of ageing, Alzheimer's disease, and other neurodegenerative conditions. *Curr Opin Neurobiol* 2016;36:43-51.

[53] Chiotis K, Saint-Aubert L, Savitcheva I, et al. Imaging in-vivo tau pathology in Alzheimer's disease with THK5317 PET in a multimodal paradigm. *Eur J Nucl Med Mol Imaging* 2016;43:1686-1699.

[54] Sheline YI, Raichle ME, Snyder AZ, et al. Amyloid Plaques Disrupt Resting State Default Mode Network Connectivity in Cognitively Normal Elderly. *Bio Psychiatry* 2010;67:584-587.

[55] Jack CR, Jr., Knopman DS, Jagust WJ, et al. Tracking pathophysiological processes in Alzheimer's disease: an updated hypothetical model of dynamic biomarkers. *Lancet Neurol* 2013;12:207-216.

[56] Brickman AM, Provenzano FA, Muraskin J, et al. Regional white matter hyperintensity volume, not hippocampal atrophy, predicts incident Alzheimer disease in the community. *Arch Neurol* 2012;69:1621-1627.

[57] Drzezga A, Becker JA, Van Dijk KRA, et al. Neuronal dysfunction and disconnection of cortical hubs in non-demented subjects with elevated amyloid burden. *Brain* 2011.

[58] Sperling RA, Johnson KA, Doraiswamy PM, et al. Amyloid deposition detected with florbetapir F 18 ((18)F-AV-45) is related to lower episodic memory performance in clinically normal older individuals. *Neurobiol Aging* 2013;34:822-831.

[59] Giorgio A, De Stefano N. Advanced Structural and Functional Brain MRI in Multiple Sclerosis. *Semin Neurol* 2016;36:163-176.

[60] Preziosa P, Rocca MA, Pagani E, et al. Structural MRI correlates of cognitive impairment in patients with multiple sclerosis: A Multicenter Study. *Hum Brain Mapp* 2016;37:1627-1644.

[61] Rocca MA, Vacchi L, Rodegher M, et al. Mapping face encoding using functional MRI in multiple sclerosis across disease phenotypes. *Brain Imaging Behav* 2016.

[62] Zhou Y, Kierans A, Kenul D, et al. Mild traumatic brain injury: longitudinal regional brain volume changes. *Radiology* 2013; 267:880-890.

[63] Tona F, Petsas N, Sbardella E, et al. Multiple sclerosis: altered thalamic resting-state functional connectivity and its effect on cognitive function. *Radiology* 2014;271:814-821.

Chapter 3

HOMOTOPIC IMAGING AND CORRELATIONS WITH NEUROCOGNITIVE TESTS IN MILD TRAUMATIC BRAIN INJURY, POST-TRAUMATIC STRESS DISORDER, MILD COGNITIVE IMPAIRMENT AND MULTIPLE SCLEROSIS

ABSTRACT

Since the interhemispheric functional integration plays an important role in communicating perceptual, cognitive, learning, attention, and information processing, more detailed clinical data on neurodegenerative and psychiatric disorders regarding brain functional homotopy and systematic analyses are needed with further validation and application. Previous studies had shown good correspondence between homotopy imaging and myelin map. The purposes of this study are to: i. examine the functional homotopic differences in the four neurodegenerative diseases including PTSD, MTBI, MCI and MS compared to controls; ii. explore the correlations between quantitative VMHC values and various neurocognitive/neuropsychological tests in patients; and iii. validate with other metrics including structural connectivity and myelin map.

Regarding the VMHC differences, PTSD patients had lower homotopic connections in the parietal, temporal, thalamic radiation and optic radiation, subcortical striatum as well as frontal white matter areas, with very mild higher homotopic connections in the small regions of vmPFC compared to controls ($P < 0.01$). Different VMHC pattern of MTBI was found with patients showing lower VMHC values in the hippocampus, bilateral dorsolateral prefrontal, temporal and occipital cortices but higher VMHC in the vmPFC and small middle cingulate regions. On the other hand, MCI patients had lower homotopic connections in the cuneus and small middle frontal regions, but higher homotopic connections in the distributed temporal, occipital, motor and parietal cortices were observed ($P < 0.01$). In MS patients, significantly lower VMHC values were found mainly in the primary cortices compared with controls, including significant reductions of regional mean VMHC values in the primary visual, somatosensory, and motor cortices (all with $P < 0.04$) in MS, with increased VMHC in the subcortical areas, including the thalamus, insula, pallidum, and cerebellum.

In terms of imaging correlates of clinical tests, the regions that had lower homotopic values in PTSD patients were associated significantly with clinical symptoms. For instance, lower homotopic values in temporal and parietal cortices, thalamic radiation and optic radiation, and significant correlations of homotopic values in these regions with CAPS. Negative correlations were found between vmPFC homotopic value and GDS, ADAS and TICS in PTSD. Significant correlations between homotopic values in frontal, temporal, occipital and parietal regions and MMSE, AFQT total as well as sub-categories such as object and spatial cognitive functionality were found additionally. In MS patients, homotopic values in dorsolateral prefrontal, cerebellum and posterior cingulate were correlated positively with both fatigue and depression scores but at opposite directions. Additional significant associations were found in multiple brain regions between homotopic values in visual, temporal, motor, frontal cortices and neurocognitive tests including executive function, verbal fluency, information processing, learning and working memory, visual-perception, and sustained attention. And finally the VMHC values in several regions including cuneus, medial prefrontal and tempo-occipital conjunction areas correlated with MS EDSS score.

INTRODUCTION

Posttraumatic stress disorder is a mental disorder that can develop after a person is exposed to a traumatic event (sometimes life-threatening), with various injury causes such as warfare or traffic accident [1]. About 3.5% of adults have PTSD in a given year, and 9% at risk lifetime (Diagnostic and Statistical Manual of Mental Disorders, DSM-V, 2013). About 20%-22% people who were diagnosed with PTSD were caused by traffic accident [2-5]. About 25% of military personnel will develop PTSD, most often chronic, with displaced persons be more affected than nondisplaced persons [2, 6]. And the overall lifetime prevalence of PTSD in U.S. combat veterans is about 6% to 31% [7, 8].

Rates of comorbid PTSD and mild traumatic brain injury (MTBI) are estimated to be about 30% for TBI positive patients [9, 10]. Depending on type of exposure and age, gender, for instance, 16% of children who had been exposed to a traumatic event had developed PTSD [11]. Risk of dementia associated with veteran PTSD is about two-fold, possibly due to the decreased cognitive reserve at age [9, 12]. Some stress-related sequelae include hippocampus damage due to chronic stress or changes in the hypothalamic-pituitary-adrenal axis inflammation due to acute stress [13-15]. Re-experiencing, avoidance and hyper-arousal are the common symptoms of PTSD based on DSM-V and International Classification of Diseases and Related health Problems (ICD-11, World Health Organization) criteria [16-19]. Over-activation of the prefrontal cortex, especially ventromedial prefrontal cortex (vmPFC), and hippocampus atrophy had been reported to be associated with these symptoms in patients [13, 20-22].

Voxel-mirrored homotopic correlation (VMHC) computes the Pearson correlation between the preprocessed time-series of each pair of symmetric interhemispheric voxels in the brain based on the resting-state (RS)-fMRI data [23, 24]. A couple of previous studies found that PTSD patients had decreased interhemispheric connectivity in the superior/middle frontal gyrus [1, 25, 26]. And VMHC in the dorsolateral prefrontal cortex was decreased that might be associated with the poor outcome of executive function in TBI patients [27, 28]. Since the interhemispheric functional integration plays an important role in communicating perceptual, cognitive, learning, attention and information processing [29, 30], more detailed clinical data on neurodegenerative and psychiatric disorders regarding brain functional homotopy and systematic analyses are needed with further validation and application [1, 23, 31, 32].

Previous studies had shown good correspondence between homotopy imaging and myelin map [33-36]. The purposes of this chapter are to: i. examine the functional homotopic differences in the four neurodegenerative diseases including PTSD, MTBI, MCI and MS compared to controls; and ii. explore the correlations between quantitative VMHC values and various clinical neurocognitive/neuropsychological tests in these patients.

METHODS

Participants and Neurocognitive/Neuropsychological Tests

Same subjects population as in previous chapter went through the homotopic myelin-related neuroimaging and neurocognitive/neuro-psychological data analysis.

For the PTSD project, several available neuropsychological questionnaires, including Mini-Mental State Examination (MMSE), Alzheimer's Disease Assessment Scale–Cognitive (ADAS-Cog), Geriatric Depression Scale (GDS), Combat Exposure Scale (CES), Telephone interview for Cognitive Status (TICS) were collected from each participant [2, 22, 37, 38]. The Armed Forces Qualification Tests (AFQT) included four categories such as vocabulary ability, object discrimination, spatial orientation and mathematics sub-scores, together with the total score, were used in this study [39-42]. In addition, all participants were assessed using a battery of neuropsychological inventory (NPI) and neurocognitive tests including the clock drawing test, the Rey auditory verbal learning test, the category fluency test, the trail making test and the Boston naming test [43-47]. Details of these neuropsychological testing scores including mean, standard error and statistical comparisons between PTSD patients and controls are listed in Table 1.

Significantly higher clinician-administered PTSD scale (CAPS) (75.4±4.9 in PTSD patients vs. 29.9±4.7 in controls; P = 0.00004; Table 1) and GDS scores (4.8±0.8 in PTSD patients vs. 1.3±0.3 in controls; P < 0.0001) in PTSD patients were observed. While other 10 tests including AFQT and cognitive tests either show the trend of worse performance or no differences between patients and controls (Table 1).

Table 1. Statistical differences of neuropsychological tests between PTSD patients and controls (mean ± standard deviation)

NP Score	Control	Patient	P-value
CAPS **	29.9 ± 4.7	75.4 ± 4.9	< 0.0001
NPI	10.7 ± 4.3	18.1 ± 8.4	0.3200
AFQT Vocabulary	20.6 ± 0.9	21.9 ± 0.8	0.3906
AFQT Object	16.8 ± 0.9	16.9 ± 1.0	0.9584
AFQT Spatial	13.4 ± 1.0	14.2 ± 1.2	0.6427
AFQT Math	16.9 ± 0.9	17.0 ± 1.5	0.9681
AFQT Total	70.8 ± 2.7	70.1 ± 3.6	0.8786
CES	13.5 ± 1.5	16.8 ± 2.2	0.2456
GDS**	1.3 ± 0.3	4.8 ± 0.8	<0.0001
MMSE	28.2 ± 0.2	27.8 ± 0.5	0.4180
TICS	34.7 ± 0.4	34.6 ± 0.8	0.8576
ADAS	11.5 ± 0.6	13.8 ± 1.4	0.0866

Significantly higher CAPS and GDS scores in patients were observed (P < 0.0001); and other tests either show the trend of worse performance or no differences.

For MS and MTBI projects, clinical assessment included two main components: neurocognitive testing results and scores from an array of established clinical symptom scales. Clinical assessment was performed within 12 hours of MR imaging for all participants, including control subjects for the two projects [23, 48]. Neurocognitive testing was performed by a trained neuropsychologist who was blinded to MR imaging results. The neurocognitive battery comprised the following tests: *(a)* the Symbol Digit Modalities Test (SDMT), a measure of information processing speed [49]; *(b)* the Digit Span subtest of the Wechsler Adult Intelligence Scale III, a measure of verbal attention, concentration, and working memory [50]; *(c)* Trail-Making Test A, which is used to assess speed and visual attention; Trail-Making Test B (TMB), a measure of mental flexibility (specifically, the ability to shift rapidly between cognitive sets) (Both Trail-Making Tests are measures of attention) [51]; *(d)* the California Verbal Learning Test (CVLT) II to assess verbal learning, immediate and delayed verbal memory [52]; *(e)* the Rey-Osterrieth Complex Figure Test (RCFT) to assess visuoperceptual ability as well as immediate and delayed visual memory [53]; and *(f)* the Paced Auditory Serial Addition Test (PASAT) with four trials; as well as *(g)* cognitive examination (CE) and *(h)* Delis-Kaplan executive function scale (D-KEFS) to assess sustained attention and concentration, working memory, executive function, and information processing ability, information speed and accuracy [54-59].

In both MTBI and MS patients, the Beck anxiety inventory and the Beck depression inventory were also performed to assess anxious and depressive symptoms separately [60, 61]. Fatigue was measured by using the fatigue severity scale [62] and subjective symptoms associated with the post-concussive state were assessed by using the post concussion symptom scale (PCSS) [63]. These test results were reported in *z* scores after standardization with the control data and were normalized with the study subject's age and education level; higher *z* scores indicate better performance [64-67]. In addition, expanded disability status scale (EDSS) [68] score of 2.47 (range, 0–6) was obtained in patients with MS.

There are significant differences between MS patients and controls in the D-KEFS for category switching ($P = 0.005$) and interference switching ($P = 0.004$), Becky depression index (BSI) ($P = 0.019$) and Fatigue severity scale ($P = 0.027$); but no significant difference for other tests including the CVLT delayed recall and D-KEFS.

As reported in our previous work, patients with MTBI demonstrated significantly higher scores on scales of depression and anxiety, as well as the PCSS, both at the initial visit and at the 1-year follow-up visits ($P<0.05$) [67]. A two-way Friedman nonparametric ANOVA with post-hoc comparison that included age and time to MR imaging after injury as covariates showed significantly increased depression scores for patients at 1-year follow-up compared with the initial visit ($P = 0.001$).

There were no differences in performance on neurocognitive tests between patients with MTBI and control subjects at initial visit. At 1-year follow-up, patients with MTBI showed improvement in performance ($P < 0.05$) on two specific neurocognitive tests (the Digit Span test and the RCFT, tests of working memory and attention) compared with initial assessment. Also in MTBI, the left rostral anterior cingulate (rAC) volume loss in patients correlated positively with longitudinal change in CVLT score over time ($r = 0.65$, $P = 0.005$) and loss of right rAC volume correlated positively with longitudinal change in PASAT trial 2 score over time ($r = 0.60$, $P = 0.01$). At 1-year follow-up, patients showed a negative correlation between left cingulate gyrus isthmus white matter (WM) volume and anxiety score on the Beck Anxiety Inventory (Spearman rank correlation $r = -0.68$, $P = 0.007$). In addition, there was a negative correlation between left cingulate gyrus isthmus WM volume and PCSS ($r = -0.65$, $P = 0.01$) [67].

Data Processing

VMHC was computed as the interhemispheric synchrony or voxel-mirrored hemispheric correlation after preprocessing of RS-fMRI, similar to the voxel-wise fcMRI computation steps. The resultant values were z-transformed (by use of the Fisher r-to-z transform) and were used for subsequent group-level analysis. We used a 2-sample Student t test to compare VMHC between the patient group and the healthy control group. The participant's age and sex were used as covariants for comparison to derive the results. Multiple comparison corrections at the cluster level were performed to the whole brain based on Gaussian random field (GRF) theory using the FSL easy thresh command (minimum $Z > 2.3$; cluster significance, $P < 0.05$, corrected) [23, 24].

The global VMHC score for each participant was obtained by the average of the VMHC z-images of each participant within the 25% gray matter mask from the FSL template for further quantification. Regional VMHC values were obtained based on the 50% and 112 total parcellation masks of the left and right hemispheric regions, with in-house developed scripts according to FSL (www.fmrib.ox.ac.uk/fsl) and Matlab software (www.mathworks.com; MathWorks, Natick, Massachusetts). These brain regions are further classified into 3 functional hierarchic subdivisions, namely primary sensory-motor, unimodal association, and heteromodal association areas [69]. Then average values of each hierarchy can be quantified as described by Stark et al. to compare between patient and control groups [29]. The primary motor and sensory cortices are engaged directly with the environment including the postcentral gyrus (somatosensory), intracalcarine cortex and occipital pole (visual), Heschl gyrus (auditory), and precentral gyrus (motor). Unimodal association areas are those regions adjacent to the primary sensory-motor cortices involved in integration of information from predominantly 1 sensory or motor technique (e.g., supramarginal gyrus, occipital fusiform gyrus). The heteromodal association areas, located primarily in the prefrontal and temporoparietal cortices, integrate information from multiple sensory and motor modalities.

Differences of homotopic images between patients including PTSD, MTBI, MCI and MS were analyzed with FSL and SPM (www.fil.ion.ucl.ak.uk) software. Statistical correlations between VMHC images and clinical tests were performed with Matlab software.

Structural connectivity data was obtained with diffusion tensor imaging (DTI) to generate mean and corpus callosum fractional anisotropy (FA) metrics, as well as to further correlate with VMHC and neuurocognitive tests [23]. As for myelin mapping, multimodal T1, T2, thickness and functional/structural MRI data from the Human Connectome Project (HCP, http://www.humanconnectomeproject.org) with an objective semi-automated neuroanatomical approach to generate 180 areas per hemisphere bounded by sharp changes in cortical architecture function, connectivity, and topography were delineated for further comparison and cross-validation [35].

RESULTS

1. Homotopy Results in PTSD, MTBI, MCI and MS

In healthy control participants, several primary cortical regions including primary visual, motor, and somatosensory cortices showed the strongest VMHC, whereas the prefrontal and temporoparietal-associated cortices and the paracingulate areas demonstrated relatively weaker VMHC. Based on voxel-wise comparison, PTSD patients had lower homotopic correlations in the thalamus, temporal, parietal and occipital cortices, and frontal white matter areas as well as thalamic radiation, optic radiation and subcortical striatum, with very mildly higher homotopic connections in the small regions of vmPFC compared to controls ($P < 0.01$) (Figure 1).

Hierarchal sub-division quantification showed PTSD patients had significantly lower VMHC values ($P < 0.01$) in several brain regions including primary and associate auditory cortices, associate somatosensory and visual cortices, as well as heteromodal paracingulate, limbic and subcortical areas (Figure 2). Detailed statistical comparison results of 112 brain regions were also listed in Table 2 ($P < 0.05$). The regions had significantly lower ($P<0.05$) VMHC in PTSD patients included bilateral superior parietal lobule, central opercular cortex and parietal opercular cortex, temporal fusiform cortex, temporal occipital fusiform, occipital fusiform gyrus, thalamus, and left caudate; with only the posterior cingulated showed higher VMHC. The most significant differences were presented in the bilateral parietal operculum cortex and bilateral occipital fusiform gyrus ($P\leq0.01$).

Hierarchal sub-division quantification showed that MTBI had much lower VMHC values in the primary visual, associate auditory and limbic areas, but higher VMHC in the primary auditory cortex, primary motor cortex, and subcortical areas compared to controls (Figure 3). Whole-brain voxel-wise comparison showed MTBI patients had lower homotopic connections in the hippocampus, bilateral dorsolateral prefrontal, temporal and occipital cortices; with higher VMHC in the vmPFC, subcortical area, motor, cuneus, and small middle cingulate regions (P < 0.01, Figure 4). 112 regional comparison showed MTBI had lower VMHC values in the bilateral planum polare, left occipital pole and right hippocampus, with higher VMHC in the bilateral accumbens compared to controls (P < 0.05) (Table 3).

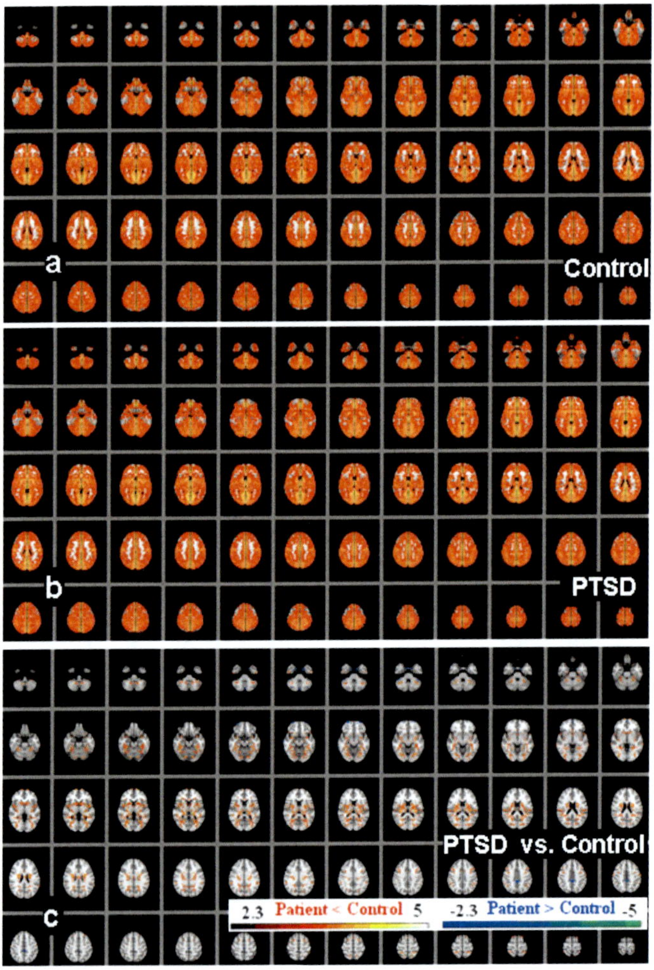

Figure 1. PTSD patients had lower homotopic connections in the thalamus, temporal, parietal occipital, and frontal white matter areas as well as thalamic radiation, optic radiation and subcortical striatum, with very mild higher homotopic connections in the small regions of vmPFC (blue color) compared to controls (P < 0.01).

Table 2. Significant regional VMHC Z-value differences with hierarchy (H) and group (R) differences between PTSD and age-matched control groups (P < 0.05)

ROI Name	Control	PTSD	Pct Diff.	P-value
L Superior Parietal Lobule H2 R2	0.5340	0.4106	-23.11	0.0223
L Central Opercular Cortex H2 R2	0.3481	0.2545	-26.89	0.0148
L Parietal Operculum Cortex H2 R2	0.3542	0.2516	-28.97	0.0080
R Superior Parietal Lobule H2 R2	0.5230	0.4203	-19.64	0.0450
R Central Opercular Cortex H2 R2	0.3506	0.2656	-24.25	0.0344
R Parietal Operculum Cortex H2 R2	0.2901	0.1807	-37.71	0.0035
L Temporal Fusiform Cortex, posterior H2 R4	0.4043	0.3031	-25.04	0.0378
L Temporal Occipital Fusiform Cortex H2 R4	0.4784	0.3119	-34.80	0.0157
L Occipital Fusiform Gyrus H2 R4	0.5566	0.4112	-26.12	0.0136
R Temporal Occipital Fusiform Cortex H2 R4	0.4367	0.2876	-34.13	0.0220
R Occipital Fusiform Gyrus H2 R4	0.5519	0.3938	-28.65	0.0089
R Cingulate Gyrus, posterior division H4	0.5584	0.6436	15.25	0.0277
L Thalamus H6	0.7955	0.6913	-13.10	0.0309
L Caudate H6	0.6656	0.5436	-18.32	0.0447
R Thalamus H6	0.7571	0.6465	-14.60	0.0238

Table 3. Significant regional VMHC Z-value differences with hierarchy (H) and group (R) between MTBI and age, education level-matched control groups (P < 0.05)

ROI Name	Control	MTBI	Pct Diff.	P-value
L Occipital Pole H1 R3	0.7505	0.6288	-16.22	0.0368
L Planum Polare H2 R6	0.4843	0.3969	-18.06	0.0422
R Planum Polare H2 R6	0.5043	0.3887	-22.93	0.0106
R Hippocampus H5	0.4214	0.2953	-29.94	0.0471
L Accumbens H6	0.5666	0.8214	44.96	0.0399
R Accumbens H6	0.5762	0.8423	46.17	0.0311

Notice that since the mean age of the MTBI population is about half to that of the PTSD population, the regional VMHC of the MTBI control is slightly different than the PTSD control group, including higher in the primary cortex but lower in the unimodal visual cortex.

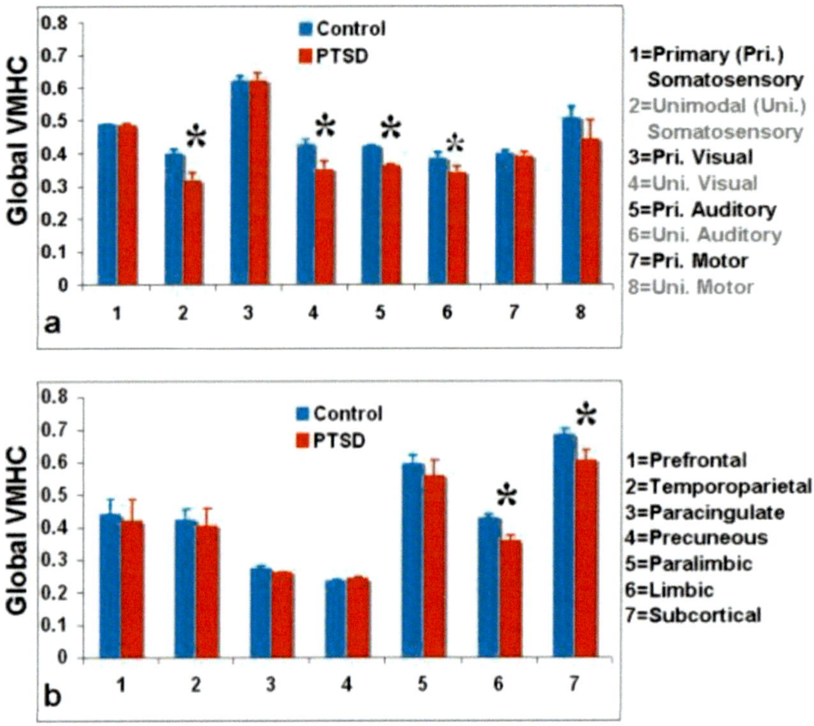

Figure 2. Bar plots showing the hierarchal regional quantification of homotopic values according to the multi-modal regional (R) classification including primary, unimodal (a) and heteromodal parcellations as well as the functional hierarchal (H) subdivision (b). Both controls and patients showed highest VMHC in the primary visual cortex following with the somatosensory cortex, similar to the myelin distribution in the brain. PTSD patients had lower VMHC values in most of brain regions including associate somatosensory and visual cortices, primary and associate auditory cortices in (a), as well as paracingulate, limbic and subcortical areas in (b).

Compared to age-matched controls, MCI patients had lower homotopic connections in the cuneus, inferior parietal lobe, and medial prefrontal cortex. Higher homotopic connections in the temporal, occipital, superior frontal, motor and parietal cortices were observed in MCI patients as well ($P < 0.01$; Figure 5). The higher VMHC in the temporal and superior frontal regions in MCI compared to controls was possibly due to more negative VMHC in the patients group with age.

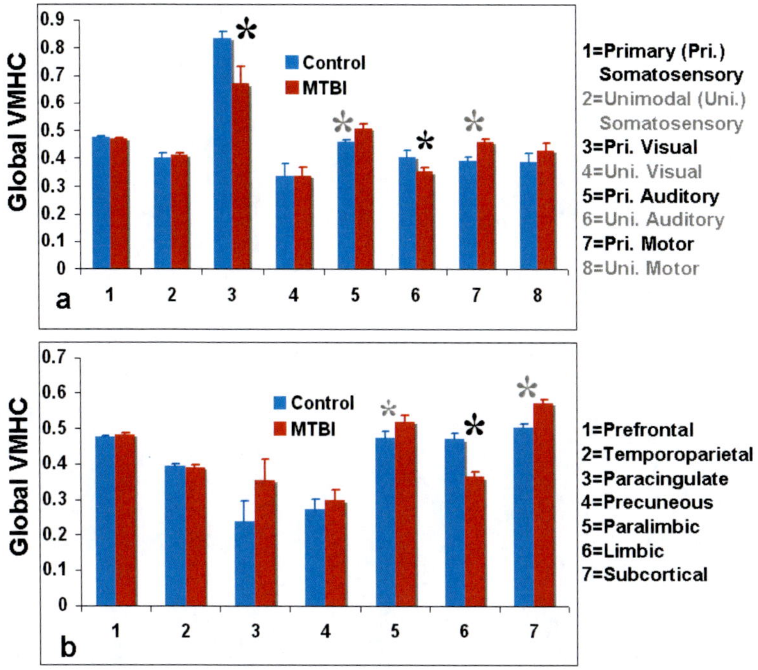

Figure 3. a: Regional hierarchal quantification of VMHC values the four primary and unimodal areas. b: Seven heteromodal prefrontal, temporo-parietal and limbic regions. MTBI had much lower VMHC values in the primary visual, associate auditory and limbic areas, but higher VMHC in the primary auditory cortex, primary motor cortex, and subcortical areas.

Table 4. Brain regions showed VMHC differences in two groups; only right side is listed due to symmetric computation between hemispheres showing significantly decreased VMHC in patients compared to controls (corrected P < 0.05, cluster size ⩾ 20) [23]

Brain Region	BA	X,Y,Z, MNI mm	Cluster size	Max. Z Score
Visual (Calcarine)	17	-10, -94, -2	905	3.83
Primary Somatosensory	1	-50, -16, 46	286	3.8
Lateral Occipital	19	-34, -74, -4	163	3.58
Middle Temporal	22	-66, -46, 8	129	4.07
Frontal Pole	11	-36, 64, -6	126	3.52
Superior Temporal	48	-54, -4, -2	93	3.88
Inferior Occipital	18	-24, -70, -16	65	3.41
Middle Occipital	37	-38, -42, -28	64	3.06
Fusiform	37	-22, -54, -14	59	3.35
Cuneus	19	-12, -82, 34	57	3.68

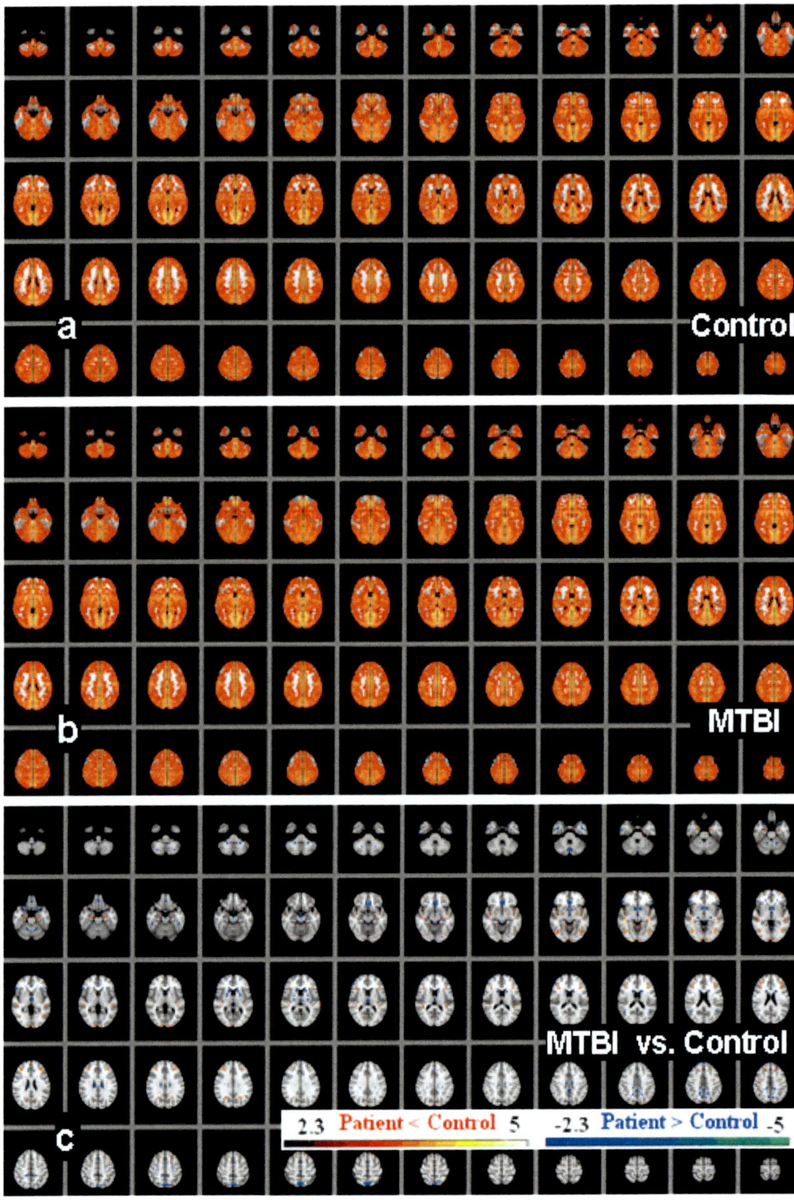

Figure 4. Compared to controls, MTBI patients showed lower homotopic connections in the hippocampus, bilateral dorsolateral prefrontal, temporal and occipital cortices; higher in the vmPFC, subcortical area, motor, cuneus and small middle cingulate regions (P<0.01).

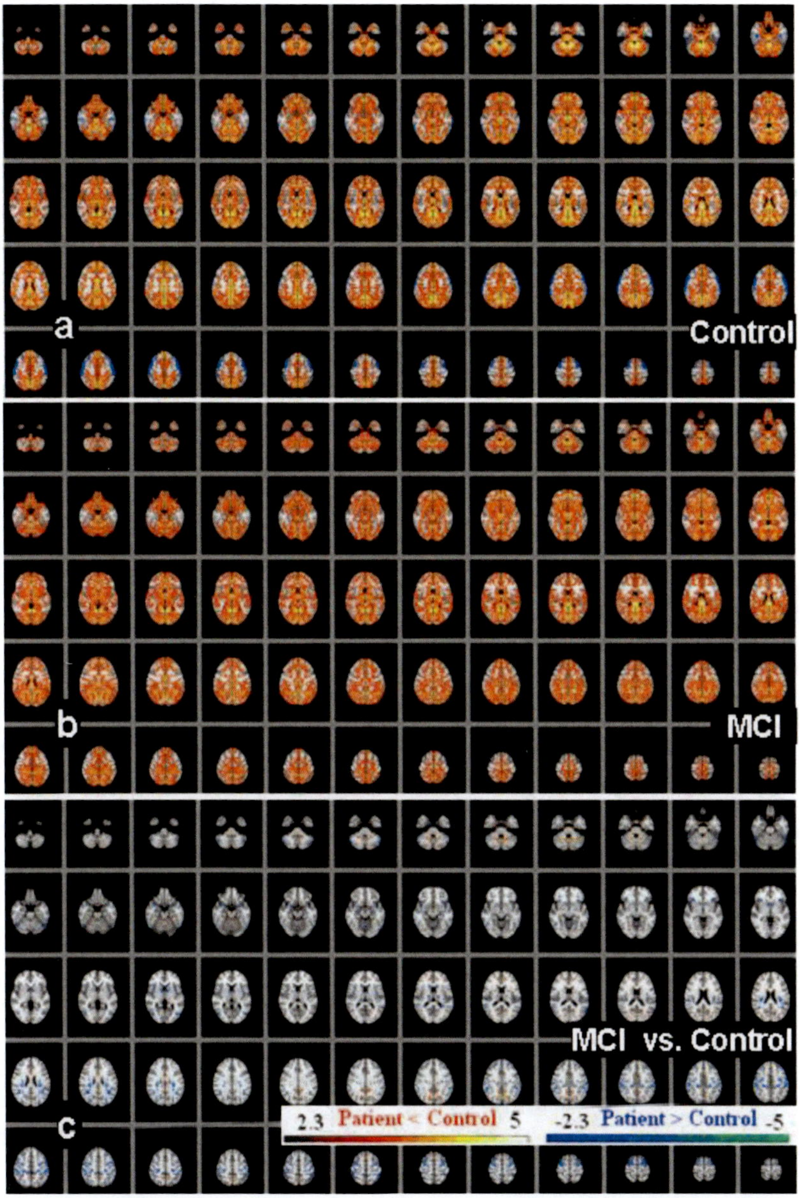

Figure 5. MCI patients had lower homotopic connections in the cuneus, inferior parietal lobe, and medial prefrontal cortex. Higher homotopic connections in the distributed regions in the temporal, superior frontal, occipital, motor and parietal cortices were observed in MCI patients compared to controls ($P < 0.01$).

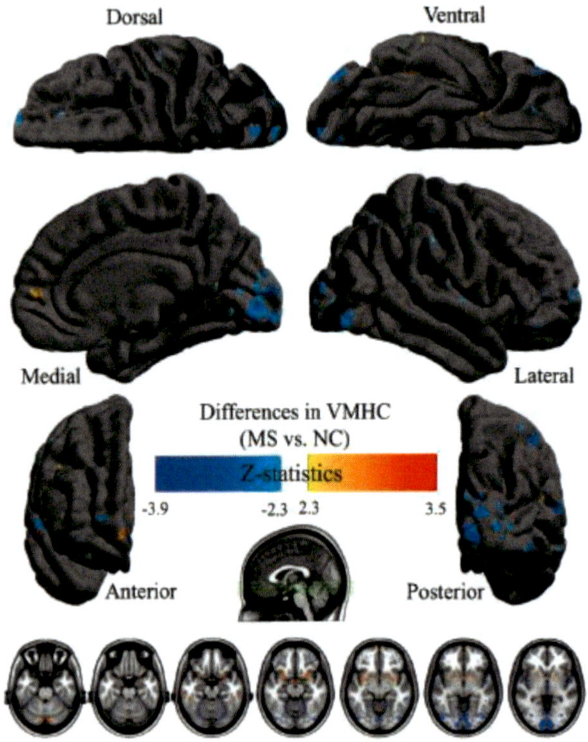

Figure 6. Comparison results of whole-brain voxel-wise VMHC maps between patients with MS and healthy control participants showed regions with significantly decreased (blue) and increased VMHC (red and yellow) in patients compared with control participants corrected with Gaussian random field theory (minimum Z > 2.3; cluster level; P < 0.05, corrected) [23].

Table 5. Brain regions showed VMHC differences in two groups; only right side is listed due to symmetric computation between hemispheres showing significantly increased VMHC in patients compared to controls (corrected P < 0.05, cluster size ⩾ 20) [23]

Brain Region	BA	X,Y,Z, MNI mm	Cluster size	Max. Z Score
Orbital frontal/Insular	48	-26, -12, -14	160	3.45
Thalamus	-	-2, -24, 12	40	3.16
Cerebellum	-	-10, -82, -26	40	3.44
Pallidum	-	-10, 4, -4	23	3.19
Inferior Temporal	20	-48, -34, -20	22	3.71

Comparison results of whole-brain voxel-wise VMHC maps between patients with MS and healthy control participants showed regions with significantly decreased VMHC in the visual, prefrontal and scattered temporal cortices and increased VMHC in the subcortical and cerebellar regions, in patients (corrected with Gaussian random field theory; minimum $Z > 2.3$; cluster level; $P < 0.05$; Figure 6) [23]. Regional interhemispheric VMHC analysis found the highest values in the visual cortex followed by the somatosensory, auditory, and motor areas in both groups. Much higher regional homotopic connectivity in the primary cortices compared with unimodal and heteromodal regions in both MS and control groups. Specifically, there was decreased VMHC within many higher-order cognitive regions, including the frontal, temporal, and occipital lobes, in patients compared with control participants (corrected $P < 0.05$). On the other hand, there was also increased VMHC in the anterior insular, thalamus, striatum, cerebellum, and inferior temporal regions in patients compared with control participants, and these regions are mainly associated with sensory processing and motor control. Detailed comparison of VMHC in different regions between the two groups is shown in Tables 4 and 5. Global mean VMHC in the MS group was decreased compared to control group ($P = 0.04$), indicating a deficit of whole-brain inter-hemispheric synchronization in the patients.

2. Correlations between Homotopy Images and Clinical Tests Including Neurocognitive and Neuropsychological Scales

a. Correlation between VMHC and Tests in PTSD Patients

Significantly negative correlations between homotopic connections and PTSD CAPS were found in regions of temporal, subcortical putamen, uncinate fasciculus, thalamic radiation, optic radiation and parietal regions. While positive correlations only existed in small regions in the cerebellum and vmPFC (Figure 7a).

On the other hand, significantly positive correlations between homotopic connections and neuropsychological inventory score were found in the hippocampus, anterior temporal, occipital, cuneus and parietal regions (Figure 7b; red color). Negative correlations only existed in small scattering regions in the cerebellum and occipital cortices. Positive correlations between homotopic connections and CES in the cerebellum, small regions in insula, anterior and middle cingulate, as well as dorsolateral and medial prefrontal cortices were found ($P < 0.01$), and negative correlations existed in small regions in inferior temporal, inferior parietal and occipital cortices (Figure 7c).

For the PTSD patients, significant positive correlations between GDS score and homotopic connections in the gyrus rectus and inferior orbitofrontal regions exited; on the other hand, negative correlations in the vmPFC, medial prefrontal and dorsolateral prefrontal cortices, as well as in the cerebellum, thalamus, superior temporal and occipital regions were found (Figure 8a).

Significant negative correlations were present between ADAS score and VMHC in large areas of orbitofrontal cortex including vmPFC, temporal cortex including hippocampus, midbrain, thalamic radiation and motor area; positive correlations existed only in the small occipital regions ($P < 0.01$; Figure 8b).

Significant positive correlations between MMSE score and homotopic connectivity in the temporal, vmPFC, occipital and angular regions, as well as dorsolateral prefrontal cortex were found (Figure 9a). As regarding AFQT total score, positive correlations with homotopic connectivity in the medial prefrontal and orbitofrontal cortices were found, as well as in the temporal cortex including hippocampus, subcortical caudate and thalamus; negative in the cerebellum, temporo-occipital conjunction, and cuneus (Figure 9b).

For the AFQT object score, positive correlations existed in the posterior temporal cortex including fusiform, cuneus, occipital cortex, posterior cingulate, medial prefrontal region; and negative correlations in the inferior temporal region, hypothalamus, motor and dorsolateral prefrontal regions (Figure 9c).

For the connection between homotopic connectivity and AFQT mathematics score, positive correlations in small regions in the angular, fusiform, vmPFC, cuneus were found; negative correlations in medial prefrontal and dorsolateral prefrontal cortices, small inferior temporal and caudate regions existed (Figure 10a).

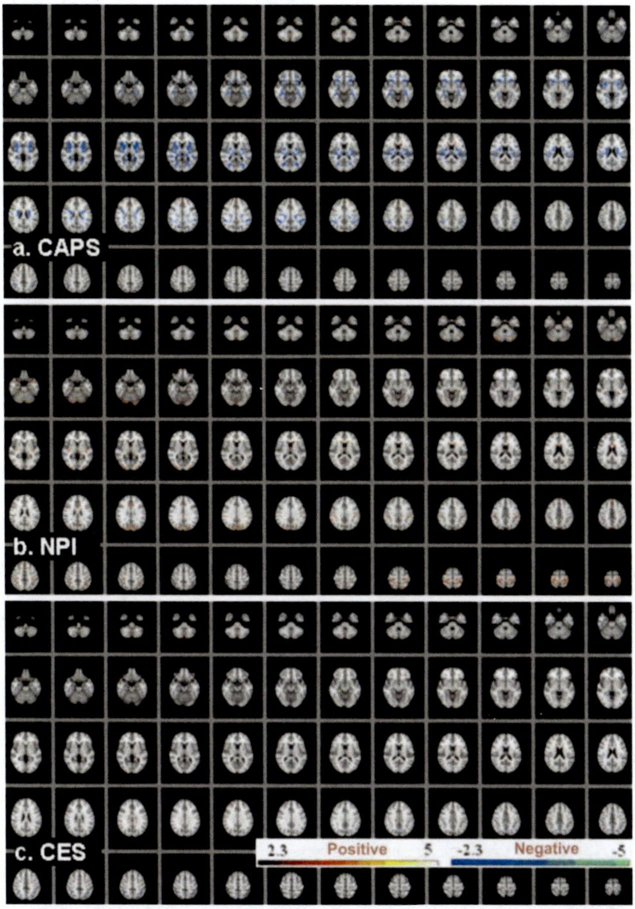

Figure 7. Significantly negative correlations between homotopic connections and PTSD CAPS were found in the temporal, subcortical putamen, uncinate fasciculus, thalamic radiation, optic radiation and parietal regions. Positive correlations only existed in small regions in the cerebellum and vmPFC ($P < 0.01$). b. Significantly positive correlations between homotopic connections and neuropsychological inventory (NPI) were found in the hippocampus, anterior temporal, occipital, cuneus and parietal/motor regions (red color). Negative correlations only existed in small scattering regions in the cerebellum and occipital cortex ($P < 0.01$). c. Positive correlations between homotopic connections and CES in the cerebellum, small regions in insula, anterior and middle cingulate, as well as dorsolateral and medial prefrontal cortices were found ($P < 0.01$), and negative correlations existed in small regions in inferior temporal, inferior parietal and occipital cortices.

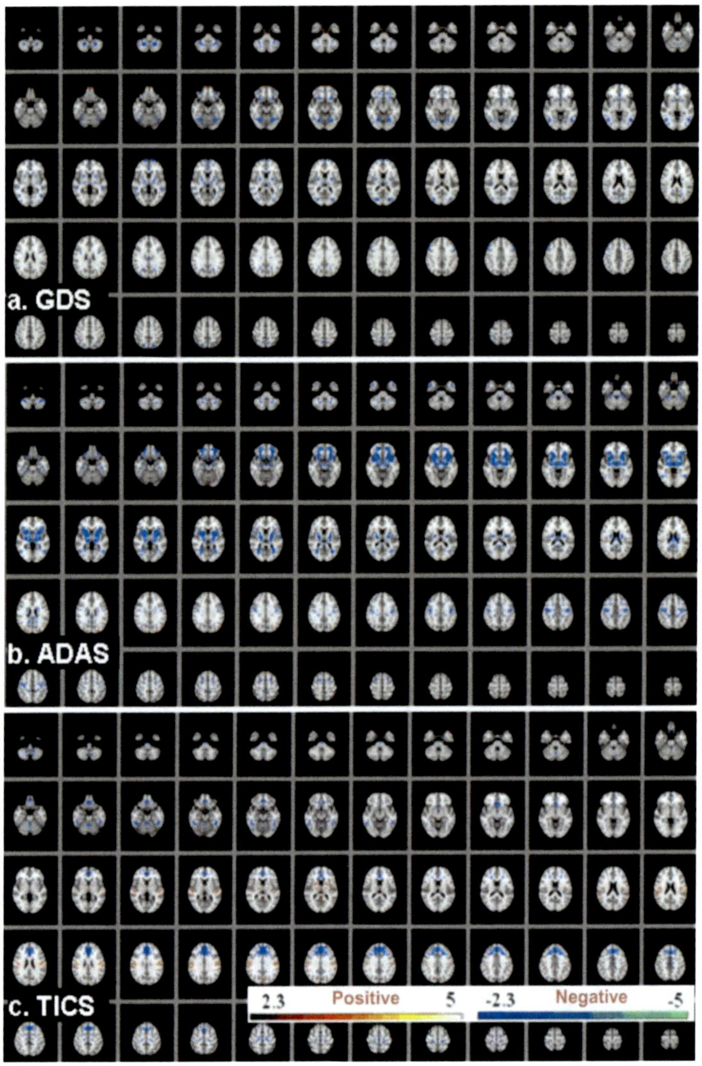

Figure 8a. GDS: significant positive correlations in the gyrus rectus and inferior orbitofrontal regions, negative correlations in the vmPFC, medial prefrontal and dorsolateral prefrontal cortices, as well as in the cerebellum, thalamus, superior temporal and occipital regions; b. ADAS: significant negative correlations in large areas of orbitofrontal cortex including vmPFC, temporal cortex including hippocampus, midbrain, thalamic radiation and motor area ($P < 0.01$); positive correlations only in small occipital region. c. TICS: significant negative correlations in vmPFC, medial prefrontal cortex, temporal region including fusiform, and small region in supplementary motor cortex; positive correlations in the temporo-parietal junction, thalamus, as well as small regions in posterior cingulate, cuneus and motor area.

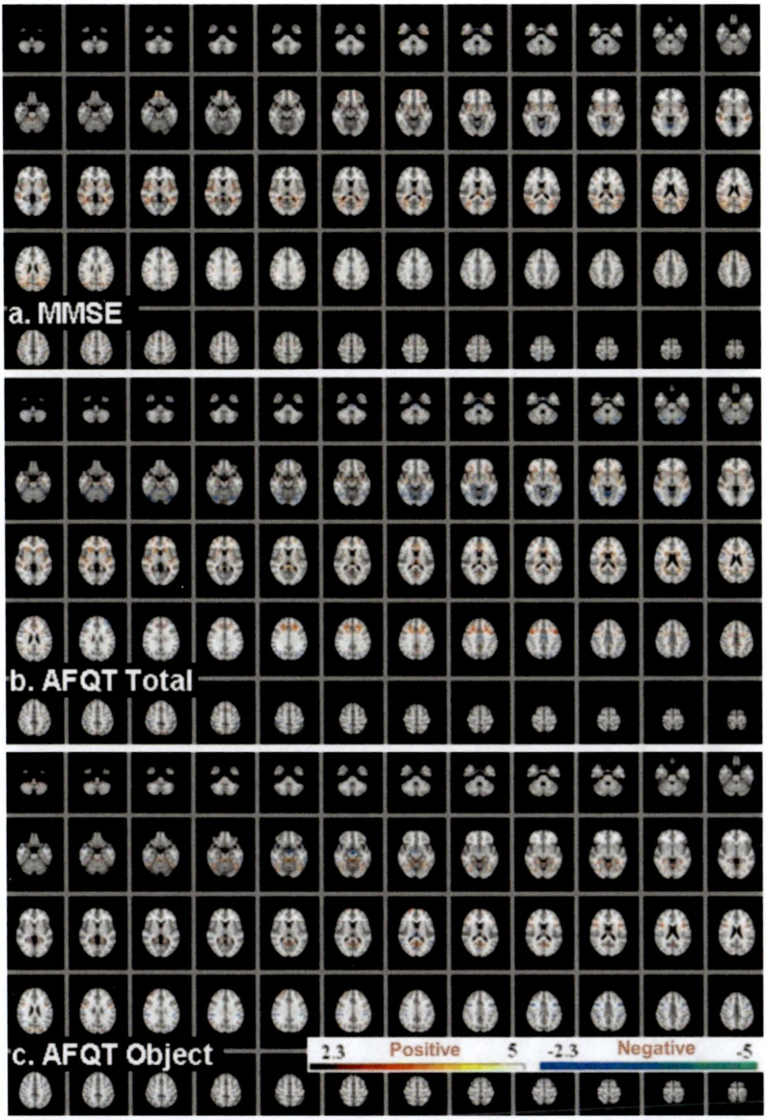

Figure 9a. MMSE: significant positive correlations in the temporal, vmPFC, occipital and angular regions, as well as dorsolateral prefrontal cortex; b. AFQT Total: positive in the medial prefrontal and orbito-prefrontal, temporal cortex including hippocampus, subcortical caudate and thalamus; negative in the cerebellum, temporo-occipital conjunction, and cuneus; c. AFQT Object: positive correlations in the posterior temporal cortex including fusiform, occipital cortex, cuneus, posterior cingulate, medial prefrontal region; negative correlations in the inferior temporal region, hypothalamus, motor and dorsolateral prefrontal regions.

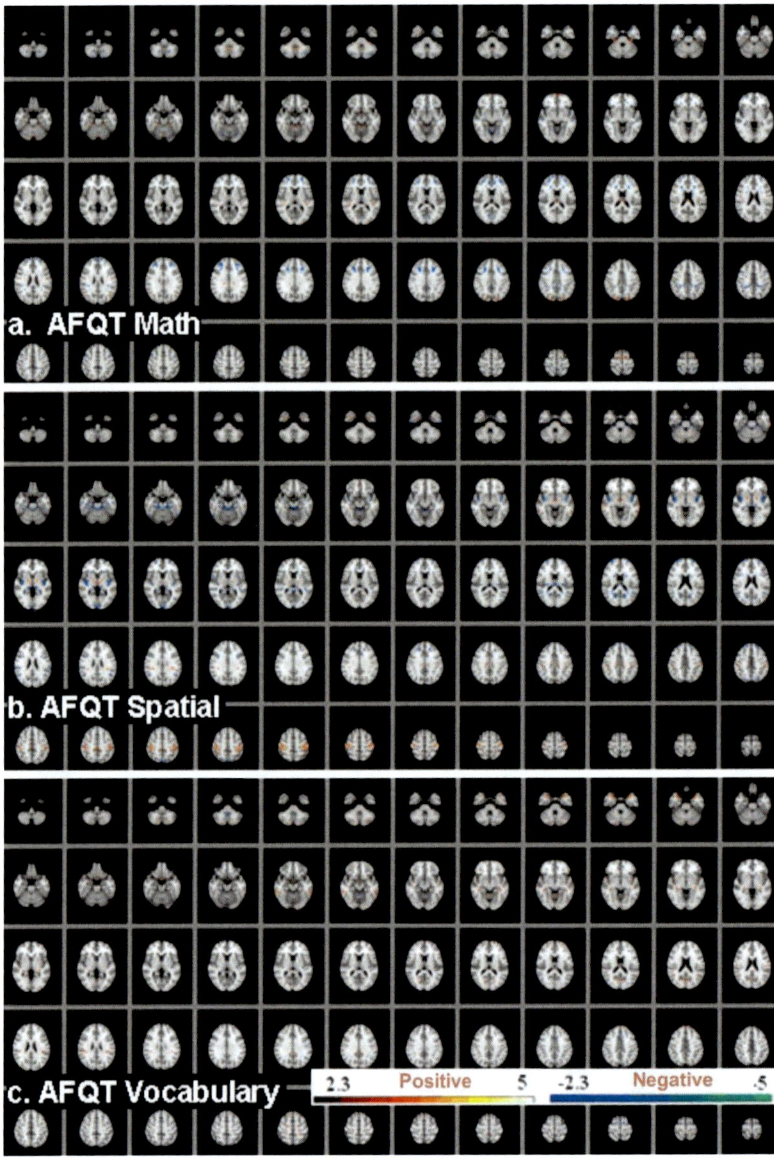

Figure 10a. AFQT Math: positive correlations in the small regions in the vmPFC, angular, fusiform and cuneus; negative in medial prefrontal and dorsolateral prefrontal cortices, small inferior temporal and caudate regions; b. AFQT Spatial: positive the motor area and inferior temporal regions as well as thalamus; negative in the small region of posterior temporal, parietal, medial frontal, insular and cuneus cortices; c. AFQT Vocabulary: positive in small regions of temporal and parietal cortices, precuneus and post-central area.

For the AFQT spatial orientation score, positive correlations with homotopic connectivity in the vmPFC, motor area and inferior temporal regions as well as thalamus, and negative correlations in the small region of posterior temporal, parietal, medial prefrontal, insular and cuneus cortices were identified (Figure 10b). For the AFQT vocabulary ability score, positive correlations with homotopic connectivity were found in small regions of temporal and parietal cortices, precuneus and post-central area (Figure 10c).

b. Correlation between VMHC and Neurocognitive Tests in MS Patients

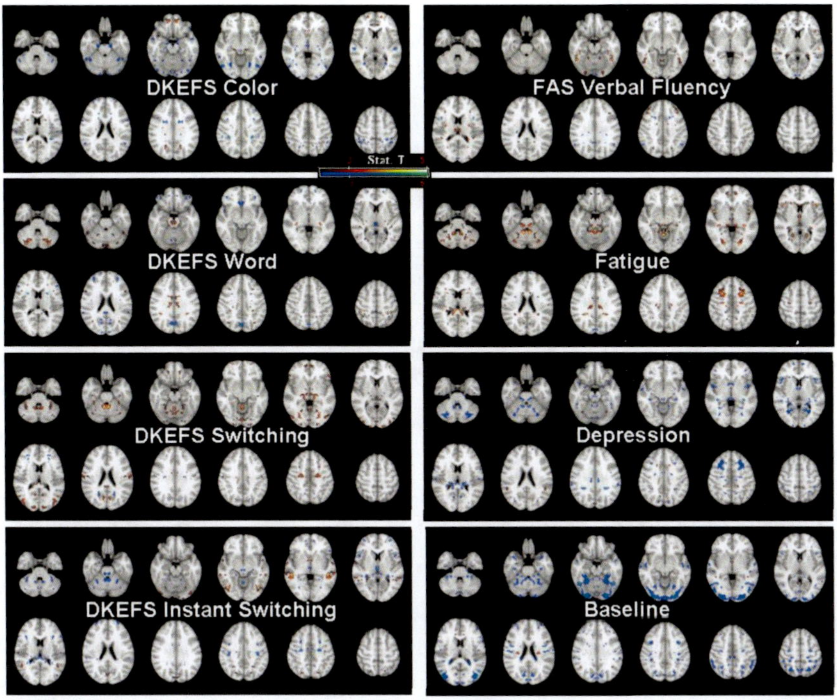

Figure 11. Dorsolateral prefrontal (DLPFC), cerebellum and posterior cingulate for Fatigue (positive) and Depression (negative), and these two symptoms had almost the same spatial associations with VMHC but at opposite correlations. V3-V4 for color, Broca's and Wernicke's areas for word processing and verbal fluency, cerebellum, vmPFC and superior temporal, visual, motor areas for mental flexibility and visual attention; dorsolateral prefrontal cortex for executive function.

In MS patients, homotopic values in dorsolateral prefrontal, cerebellum and posterior cingulate were correlated positively with Fatigue symptom score ($P < 0.01$) (Figure 11). Same spatial associations were found between VMHC image and depression symptom score but with negative correlations. Other significant correlations included between homotopic values in visual cortex including V3-V4 and color-related attention and neurocognitive scores of executive function; between VMHC at Broca's and Wernicke's areas and word processing and verbal fluency, cerebellum; between vmPFC and superior temporal, visual, motor areas and mental flexibility and visual attention; as well as between dorsolateral prefrontal cortex and executive function. Homotopic values in orbitofrontal, medial and dorsolateral prefrontal cortices and cuneus correlated with scores of information processing, working memory and attention; and VMHC of visual cortex, cerebellum and medial prefrontal cortex correlated with scores of visual-perception, sustained attention and executive function (Figure 12).

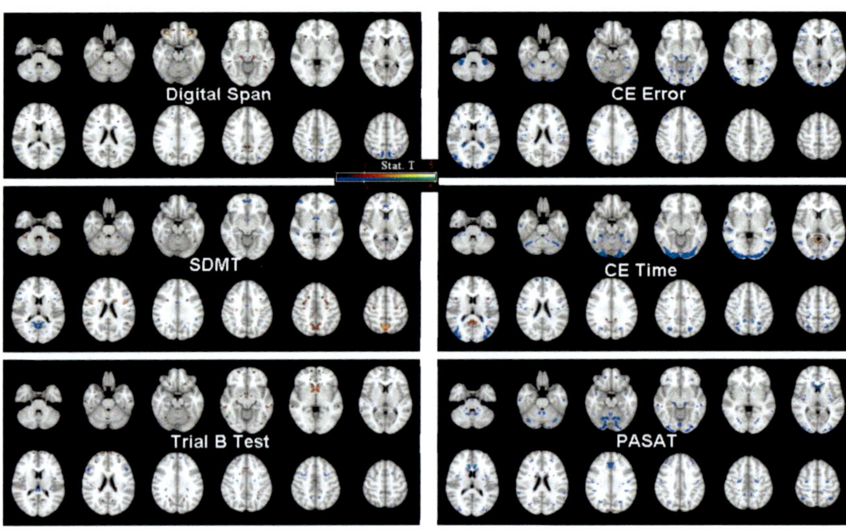

Figure 12. Orbitofrontal, medial and dorsolateral prefrontal cortices and cuneus for information processing accuracy and time, working memory and executive function existed; while visual cortex, cerebellum, temporal and medial prefrontal cortices for visual-perception, auditory and sustained attention.

Negative correlations between homotopic values in the anterior temporal and superior temporal and the delayed recall that might encode memory information were found, same for the Broca's and orbitofrontal areas for immediate recall; temporal cortex, posterior cingulate, dorsolateral and medial prefrontal regions for learning and memory functionality (Figure 13).

Covariance analysis of VMHC and EDSS score showed a few focused regions correlated significantly with the EDSS score in MS patients ($P < 0.01$); including the premotor, temporo-occipital and dorsolateral prefrontal areas, which are usually activated for visual motion perception, motor function and executive function processing (Figure 14).

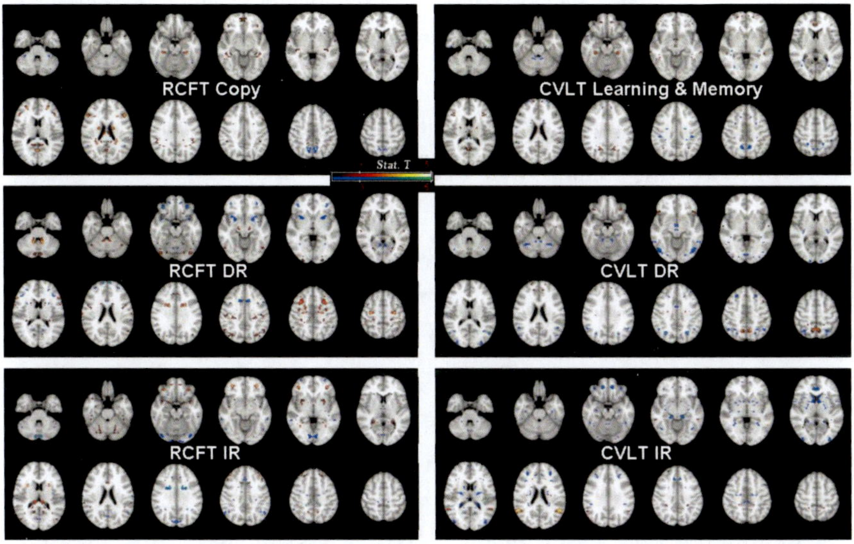

Figure 13. Significant correlations in the anterior and superior temporal segments for the delayed recall that might encode memory information functionality, Broca's and orbitofrontal areas for immediate recall; temporal cortex including hippocampus, posterior cingulate, dorsolateral and medial prefrontal regions as well as Wernicke's area for executive function, verbal learning and memory recall.

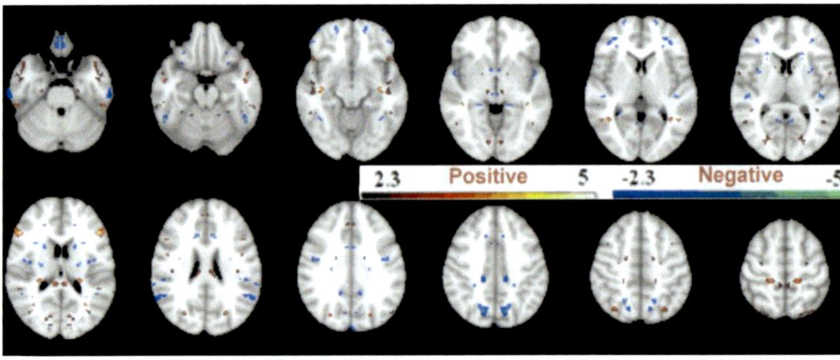

Figure 14. Significant correlation map between VMHC images and EDSS scores in MS patients ($P < 0.01$, $|T| > 2.3$). Negative correlations (blue color) included cuneus, unimodal auditory cortex (possible Wernicke's area), vmPFC, medial prefrontal, inferior temporal and motor areas; positive correlations were mainly in the medial temporal, dorsolateral frontal, premotor and primary visual cortices.

3. Validation between VMHC and Structural Connectivity, Myelin Mapping Based on Connectome

The global VMHC correlates moderately with the average fractional anisotropy (FA, a measurement for structural connectivity based on MRI DTI) of the entire corpus callosum (CC, largest interhemispheric connecting fiber) for all participants in both groups ($r = 0.3$; $P = 0.03$) [23]. A significant positive correlation was also found between the average regional VMHC in the occipital cortex and mean FA values of CC segment 5 corresponding to occipital projections ($r = 0.43$; $P = 0.037$). Furthermore, consistent with the functional connectivity correlational results, there were significantly positive correlations ($P<0.05$) between the mean FA value, primarily in the CC segment CC1/CC2/CC5, and the RCFT immediate and delayed-recalled scores in the MS patients and controls; also between the FA and the neurocognitive Trail-making test B score in the MS patients (Table 6).

Table 6. Correlation between FA in the corpus callosum (CC) and cognitive tests

DTI FA vs. Cognitive	FA of CC1 & RCFT-IR	FA of CC1 & RCFT-DR	FA of CC2 & RCFT-IR	FA of CC2 & RCFT-IR	FA of CC5 & Trail B
MS	**r = 0.674 P = 0.012**	**r = 0.721 P = 0.005**	**r = 0.700 P = 0.008**	**r = 0.606 P = 0.028**	**r = 0.564, P = 0.045**
Control	r = 0.578 P = 0.063	**r = 0.652 P = 0.030**	**r = 0.612 P = 0.046**	r = 0.526 P = 0.097	r = 0.553 P = 0.078

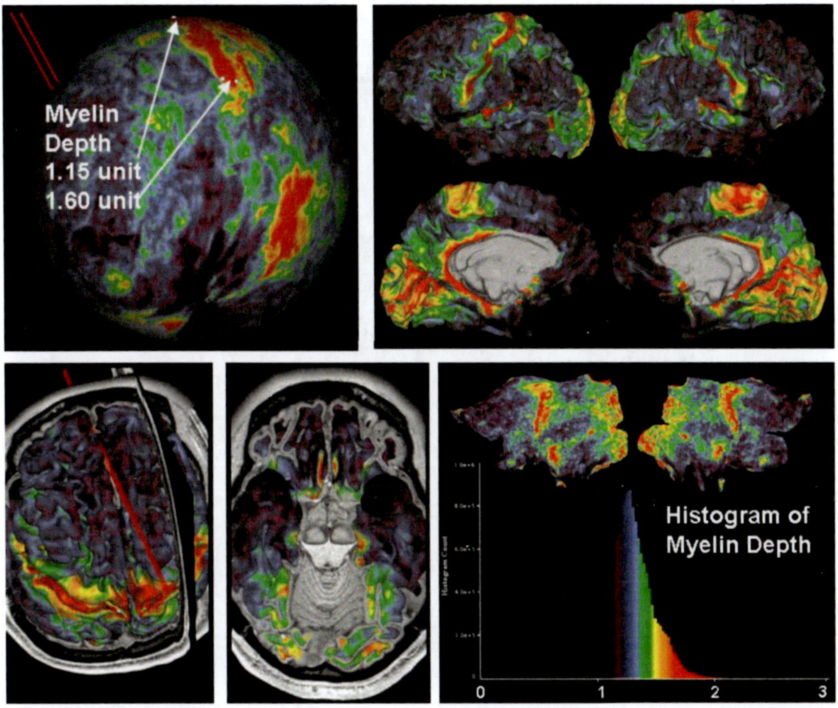

Figure 15. Myelin map with multi-band connectome technique. 3D surface, rendering and flat maps demonstrate the myelin depth (scale to the minimum 1 in brain) distribution in the brain. Highest density of myelin are shown in the visual cortex, followed by the somatosensory cortex and cingulum as well as temporal-parietal junctions, lowest in the heteromodal prefrontal and anterior temporal cortices. Myelin stripes in the visual and somatosensory cortices can be appreciated. The histogram of myelin depth revealed about 1.3 unit average with a maximum of ~2 units.

Based on the connectome data (http://www.humanconnectome.org), highest density of myelin are shown in the visual cortex, followed by the somatosensory cortex and cingulum as well as temporo-parietal junction, lowest in the heteromodal prefrontal and anterior temporal cortices. Myelin stripes in the visual and somatosensory cortices can be appreciated (Figure 15). The histogram of myelin depth revealed about 1.3 unit average with a maximum of ~2 units. And relatively symmetric left and right hemispheric myelin maps and robust spatial distribution pattern were found for each participant (Figure 16).

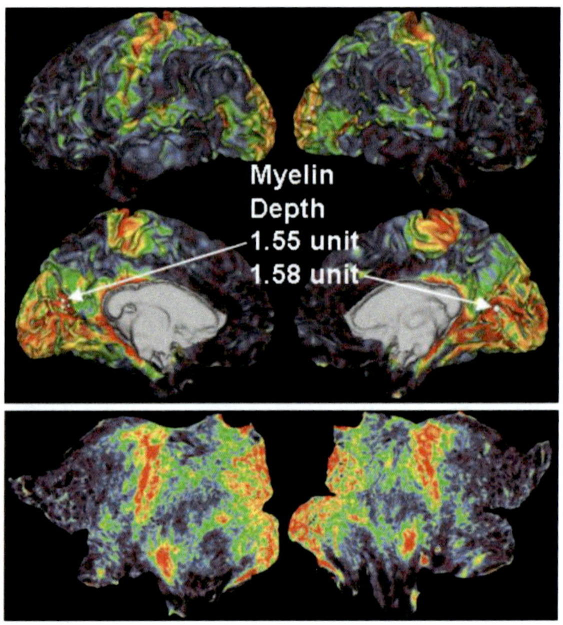

Figure 16. Myelin map from another representative participant, showing relatively symmetric and consistent left and right hemispheric maps, with similar distribution pattern as in Figure 15.

Demyelination is the loss of myelin sheath and is one of the hallmarks of neurodegenerative autoimmune diseases such as MS. The myelin map and VMHC quantification agree with each other in the regional distributions including highest in the visual and somatosensory cortices; and have significant aging effects [70]. Also both metrics measure the distance-based conductivity and reflect primarily MRI T2-based effects [36]. As expected, the structural conductivity facilitation of myelin and inter-hemispheric functional coordination of VMHC have similar spatial correspondence.

DISCUSSION

Our results indicated that PTSD patients had significantly lower homotopic connections in the parietal, temporal, thalamic radiation and optic radiation, subcortical striatum as well as frontal white matter areas, accompanied with higher vmPFC VMHC compared to controls. MTBI patients also showed lower VMHC values in the hippocampus, bilateral dorsolateral prefrontal, temporal and occipital cortices, but higher in the vmPFC, subcortical area, motor, cuneus and small middle cingulate regions. In contrast to MTBI patients, PTSD patients had more lower-VMHC in the parietal and occipital areas, but less compensational regions in the subcortical accumbens area and motor cortex, possibly due to distorted neural activations caused by re-experiencing and sustained synchrony in PTSD. On the other hand, MCI patients had lower homotopic connections in the cuneus and DMN regions including medial prefrontal and inferior parietal cortices, but higher homotopic connections in the distributed temporal, occipital, motor and parietal cortices compared to controls. These lower interhemispheric regions were consistent with the DMN deficits observed in MCI and early AD [71, 72]. In MS patients, significantly lower VMHC values were found mainly in the primary visual, somatosensory, and motor cortices. Dysfunction of these regions is responsible for the sensory, movement, or memory deficits in MS patients [23]. Similar to the MCI patients, increased VMHC in the subcortical areas, including the thalamus, insula, pallidum, and cerebellum in MS patients compared with control participants were observed additionally. Both controls and PTSD/MTBI/MS patients showed highest VMHC in the primary visual cortex following with the somatosensory cortex, similar to the myelin distribution in the brain, and presented relatively aging effects of VMHC with lower VMHC in elderly PTSD controls and patients than MTBI adult cohort [34, 73].

Many of the increased VMHC regions in MS patients are connected via the subcortical connections such as the thalamus projections or other interhemispheric connections such as anterior/posterior commissure for inferior temporal connections or corticospinal tracts. These noncallosal interhemispheric homotopic increases are assumed to compensate for the decreased interhemispheric coordination when transcallosal function is impaired in MS. The disruption of the transcallosal inhibitory mechanism could also lead to greater activation in these regions. Higher vmPFC VMHC in MTBI and PTSD patients was consistent with the functional hyperactivity in post-trauma patients [74-76]. Higher VMHC in the distributed parietal, motor and frontal regions in MCI patients indicated possible age- and memory-related compensation as well as the reduction of some resting-state functional coordination networks. The VMHC values in some of these regions such as parietal, motor and temporal regions also had significant associations with memory scores such as ADAS and MMSE.

The regions that had lower homotopic values in PTSD patients were associated significantly with clinical symptoms, including especially higher CAPS and GDS in patients. For instance, lower homotopic values in the temporal and parietal cortices, thalamic radiation and optic radiation, subcortical striatum and frontal white matter areas, and significant correlations of homotopic values in these regions with CAPS. These regions including vmPFC, parietal, temporal and thalamus with abnormal interhemispheric integral function (measured via VMHC) might contribute to the worse clinical symptoms including depression and stress in PTSD patients. Negative correlations were found between vmPFC homotopic value and AFQT, ADAS and TICS as well; with higher vmPFC homotopic value in PTSD compared to controls. Significant correlations between homotopic values in other frontal, temporal, occipital and parietal regions and MMSE, AFQT total as well as sub-categories such as object discrimination and spatial orientation cognitive functionality were found additionally. Taken together, our VMHC imaging results suggested higher sensitivity of this imaging metric for measuring brain dysfunction in response to injuries as well as detecting brain regions associated with clinical symptoms and cognitive function [77-80].

In MS patients, homotopic values in dorsolateral prefrontal and posterior cingulate cortices were correlated significantly with both fatigue and depression scores but at largely opposite directions. Mutual interactions of depression and fatigue were the common neuropsychological symptoms that influence the quality of life in MS patients in addition to the EDSS [81, 82]. Multiple regional significant associations between VMHC and cognitive tests were found including between homotopic values in visual, temporal, motor, frontal cortices and scores of executive function, verbal fluency, information processing, working memory and attention, visual-perception, sustained attention and concentration. In addition, significant relation between homotopic changes and corpus callosum microstructural changes suggests that, as callosal degeneration increases, the functional homotopy decreases, which may be indicative of inefficient callosal transmission in patients, especially the prefrontal, motor and visual cortices. Consistent with other functional map metrics, the VMHC values in several regions including cuneus, medial prefrontal and temporo-occipital conjunction areas correlated with MS EDSS score [83, 84].

Disruption of interhemispheric functional connectivity had been reported in more psychiatric diseases including depression and insomnia [85-90]. Consistent with previous functional results [36, 90, 91], we had found abnormal VMHC patterns in the four neurodegenerative diseases and their associations with neuropsychological tests. And our results also validated the similarities between VMHC and structural connectivity with significant correlations between VMHC and corpus callosum FA; as well as agreement between VMHC and myelin maps. Both the VMHC and myelin imaging could provide future cross-validation tools for examining more neurodegeneration and neuroregeneration processes, such as myelin development in adolescents and neuroinflammation in the MS or AD with better spatial resolution using higher magnetic field for more accurate diagnosis [36, 92-95]. In addition to the conventional reports of brain function and cognitive correlates [23, 96-99], our quantitative regional and voxel-wise results in this work extend further with multi-feature and more advanced imaging technique.

Conclusion

In summary, we had reported significant differences of interhemispheric correlations in patients with neurodegenerative diseases including PTSD, MTBI, MS and MCI compared to controls based on homotopic imaging results. And the neural underpins of clinical data including neurocognitive tests and symptoms using homotopic data were illustrated in both PTSD and MS patients. Our results indicate that the VMHC fMRI technique developed in this book could be used as a quantitative and accurate diagnosis tool to identify disease alterations in brain as well as to elucidate neurobiological, functional and microstructural connections of the clinical symptoms and neurocognitive scales of patients.

References

[1] Dean KR, Hammamieh R, Mellon SH, et al. Multi-omic biomarker identification and validation for diagnosing warzone-related post-traumatic stress disorder. *Mol Psychiatry* 2019.

[2] Weiner MW, Veitch DP, Hayes J, et al. Effects of traumatic brain injury and posttraumatic stress disorder on Alzheimer's disease in veterans, using the Alzheimer's Disease Neuroimaging Initiative. *Alzheimers Dement* 2014;10:S226-235.

[3] Dai W, Liu A, Kaminga AC, et al. Prevalence of acute stress disorder among road traffic accident survivors: a meta-analysis. *BMC Psychiatry* 2018;18:188.

[4] Lin W, Gong L, Xia M, Dai W. Prevalence of posttraumatic stress disorder among road traffic accident survivors: A PRISMA-compliant meta-analysis. *Medicine* (Baltimore) 2018;97:e9693.

[5] Liu Q, Jiang M, Yang Y, et al. Prevalence of Posttraumatic Stress Disorder (PTSD) and Its Correlates Among Junior High School Students at 53 Months After Experiencing an Earthquake. *Disaster Med Public Health Prep* 2019;13:414-418.

[6] Wu X, Kaminga AC, Dai W, et al. The prevalence of moderate-to-high posttraumatic growth: A systematic review and meta-analysis. *J Affect Disord* 2019;243:408-415.

[7] Richardson LK, Frueh BC, Acierno R. Prevalence estimates of combat-related post-traumatic stress disorder: critical review. *Aust N Z J Psychiatry* 2010;44:4-19.

[8] Smith TC, Jacobson IG, Hooper TI, et al. Health impact of US military service in a large population-based military cohort: findings of the Millennium Cohort Study, 2001-2008. *BMC Public Health* 2011;11:69.

[9] Yaffe K, Vittinghoff E, Lindquist K, et al. Posttraumatic stress disorder and risk of dementia among US veterans. *Arch Gen Psychiatry* 2010;67:608-613.

[10] Zhou Y, Cao Z, Yang M, et al. Comorbid generalized anxiety disorder and its association with quality of life in patients with major depressive disorder. *Sci Rep* 2017;7:40511.

[11] Kavanaugh BC, Dupont-Frechette JA, Jerskey BA, Holler KA. Neurocognitive deficits in children and adolescents following maltreatment: Neurodevelopmental consequences and neuropsychological implications of traumatic stress. *Appl Neuropsychol Child* 2017;6:64-78.

[12] Jowett S, Karatzias T, Albert I. Multiple and interpersonal trauma are risk factors for both post-traumatic stress disorder and borderline personality disorder: A systematic review on the traumatic backgrounds and clinical characteristics of comorbid post-traumatic stress disorder/borderline personality disorder groups versus single-disorder groups. *Psychol Psychother* 2019.

[13] Van Boven RW, Harrington GS, Hackney DB, et al. Advances in neuroimaging of traumatic brain injury and posttraumatic stress disorder. *J Rehabil Res Dev* 2009;46:717-757.

[14] Vasterling JJ, Duke LM, Brailey K, Constans JI, Allain AN, Jr., Sutker PB. Attention, learning, and memory performances and intellectual resources in Vietnam veterans: PTSD and no disorder comparisons. *Neuropsychology* 2002;16:5-14.

[15] Hoffman AN, Taylor AN. Stress reactivity after traumatic brain injury: implications for comorbid post-traumatic stress disorder. *Behav Pharmacol* 2019;30:115-121.

[16] Astur RS, St Germain SA, Tolin D, Ford J, Russell D, Stevens M. Hippocampus function predicts severity of post-traumatic stress disorder. *Cyberpsychol Behav* 2006;9:234-240.

[17] Dunkley BT, Wong SM, Jetly R, Wong JK, Taylor MJ. Post-traumatic stress disorder and chronic hyperconnectivity in emotional processing. *Neuroimage Clin* 2018;20:197-204.

[18] Friedman MJ, Resick PA, Bryant RA, Brewin CR. Considering PTSD for DSM-V. *Depress Anxiety* 2011;28:750-769.

[19] Jones T, Moller MD. Implications of hypothalamic-pituitary-adrenal axis functioning in posttraumatic stress disorder. *J Am Psychiatr Nurses Assoc* 2011;17:393-403.

[20] Lanius RA, Bluhm R, Lanius U, Pain C. A review of neuroimaging studies in PTSD: heterogeneity of response to symptom provocation. *J Psychiatr Res* 2006;40:709-729.

[21] Patel R, Spreng RN, Shin LM, Girard TA. Neurocircuitry models of posttraumatic stress disorder and beyond: a meta-analysis of functional neuroimaging studies. *Neurosci Biobehav Rev* 2012;36:2130-2142.

[22] Weiner MW, Harvey D, Hayes J, et al. Effects of traumatic brain injury and posttraumatic stress disorder on development of Alzheimer's disease in Vietnam Veterans using the Alzheimer's Disease Neuroimaging Initiative: Preliminary Report. *Alzheimers Dement* (N Y) 2017;3:177-188.

[23] Zhou Y, Milham M, Zuo XN, et al. Functional homotopic changes in multiple sclerosis with resting-state functional MR imaging. *AJNR Am J Neuroradiol* 2013;34:1180-1187.
[24] Zuo XN, Kelly C, Di Martino A, et al. Growing together and growing apart: regional and sex differences in the lifespan developmental trajectories of functional homotopy. *J Neurosci* 2010;30:15034-15043.
[25] Chen S, Dong D, Jackson T, Su Y, Chen H. Altered frontal inter-hemispheric resting state functional connectivity is associated with bulimic symptoms among restrained eaters. *Neuropsychologia* 2016;81:22-30.
[26] Sun YW, Hu H, Wang Y, et al. Inter-hemispheric functional and anatomical connectivity abnormalities in traffic accident-induced PTSD: a study combining fMRI and DTI. *J Affect Disord* 2015;188:80-88.
[27] Rigon A, Duff MC, McAuley E, Kramer AF, Voss MW. Is Traumatic Brain Injury Associated with Reduced Inter-Hemispheric Functional Connectivity? A Study of Large-Scale Resting State Networks following Traumatic Brain Injury. *J Neurotrauma* 2016;33:977-989.
[28] Zhou Y, Tian M, Wang HD, et al. Activation of the Nrf2-ARE signal pathway after blast induced traumatic brain injury in mice. *Int J Neurosci* 2019;129:801-807.
[29] Stark DE, Margulies DS, Shehzad ZE, et al. Regional variation in interhemispheric coordination of intrinsic hemodynamic fluctuations. *J Neurosci* 2008;28:13754-13764.
[30] Varma G, Duhamel G, de Bazelaire C, Alsop DC. Magnetization transfer from inhomogeneously broadened lines: A potential marker for myelin. *Magn Reson Med* 2015;73:614-622.
[31] Luo X, Li K, Jia YL, et al. Abnormal of inter-hemispheric functional connectivity in elderly subjects with overweight/obesity. *Obes Res Clin Pract* 2018;12:555-561.

[32] Yang H, Bai L, Zhou Y, et al. Increased inter-hemispheric resting-state functional connectivity in acute lacunar stroke patients with aphasia. *Exp Brain Res* 2017;235:941-948.

[33] Abdollahi RO, Kolster H, Glasser MF, et al. Correspondences between retinotopic areas and myelin maps in human visual cortex. *Neuroimage* 2014;99:509-524.

[34] Fracasso A, van Veluw SJ, Visser F, et al. Lines of Baillarger in vivo and ex vivo: Myelin contrast across lamina at 7T MRI and histology. *Neuroimage* 2016;133:163-175.

[35] Glasser MF, Smith SM, Marcus DS, et al. The Human Connectome Project's neuroimaging approach. *Nat Neurosci* 2016;19:1175-1187.

[36] Zhou Y. *Neuroimaging in Multiple Sclerosis.* Nova Science Publishers 2017.

[37] Mohamed AZ, Cumming P, Srour H, et al. Amyloid pathology fingerprint differentiates post-traumatic stress disorder and traumatic brain injury. *Neuroimage Clin* 2018;19:716-726.

[38] Mohamed AZ, Cumming P, Gotz J, Nasrallah F, Department of Defense Alzheimer's Disease Neuroimaging I. Tauopathy in veterans with long-term posttraumatic stress disorder and traumatic brain injury. *Eur J Nucl Med Mol Imaging* 2019;46:1139-1151.

[39] Hyams KC. Mental health screening before troop deployment: is not supported by current evidence. *BMJ* 2006;333:979-980.

[40] Karp JF, Rudy T, Weiner DK. Persistent pain biases item response on the Geriatric Depression Scale (GDS): preliminary evidence for validity of the GDS-PAIN. *Pain Med* 2008;9:33-43.

[41] Morris JC. The Clinical Dementia Rating (CDR): current version and scoring rules. *Neurology* 1993;43:2412-2414.

[42] Morris MC, Compas BE, Garber J. Relations among posttraumatic stress disorder, comorbid major depression, and HPA function: a systematic review and meta-analysis. *Clin Psychol Rev* 2012;32:301-315.

[43] Amen DG, Raji CA, Willeumier K, et al. Functional Neuroimaging Distinguishes Posttraumatic Stress Disorder from Traumatic Brain

Injury in Focused and Large Community Datasets. *PLoS One* 2015;10:e0129659.

[44] Foa EB, Meadows EA. Psychosocial treatments for posttraumatic stress disorder: a critical review. *Annu Rev Psychol* 1997;48:449-480.

[45] Folstein MF, Folstein SE, McHugh PR. "Mini-mental state". A practical method for grading the cognitive state of patients for the clinician. *J Psychiatr Res* 1975;12:189-198.

[46] Kushner MG, Riggs DS, Foa EB, Miller SM. Perceived controllability and the development of posttraumatic stress disorder (PTSD) in crime victims. *Behav Res Ther* 1993;31:105-110.

[47] Skinner J, Carvalho JO, Potter GG, et al. The Alzheimer's Disease Assessment Scale-Cognitive-Plus (ADAS-Cog-Plus): an expansion of the ADAS-Cog to improve responsiveness in MCI. *Brain Imaging Behav* 2012;6:489-501.

[48] Zhou Y, Milham MP, Lui YW, et al. Default-mode network disruption in mild traumatic brain injury. *Radiology* 2012;265:882-892.

[49] Smith A. *Symbol Digit Modalities Test Manual.* Los Angeles: Western Psychological Services 1973.

[50] Wechsler D. *Wechsler Adult Intelligence Scale-III.* New York: The Psychological Corporation 1985.

[51] Reitan R. *Trail Making Test: Manual for Administration and Scoring.* Ariz: Reitan Neuropsychology Laboratory 1992.

[52] Delis DC, Kramer JH, Kaplan E, Ober BA. *California Verbal Learning Test.* Adult Version. Manual (2nd edition). San Antonio, TX: The Psychological Corporation. 2000.

[53] Meyers JE, Meyers KR. *Rey Complex Figure Test and Recognition Trial: Professional manual.* Odessa, FL: Psychological Assessment Resources, Inc. 1995.

[54] Cicerone KD, Azulay J. Diagnostic utility of attention measures in postconcussion syndrome. *Clin Neuropsychol* 2002;16:280-289.

[55] Gronwall D, Wrightson P. Delayed recovery of intellecutal function after minor head injury. *Lancet* 1974;2:605-609.

[56] Frisch C, Rosenblum S. Reliability and validity of the executive function and occupational routines scale (EFORTS). *Res Dev Disabil* 2014;35:2148-2157.

[57] Kamradt JM, Ullsperger JM, Nikolas MA. Executive function assessment and adult attention-deficit/hyperactivity disorder: tasks versus ratings on the Barkley deficits in executive functioning scale. *Psychol Assess* 2014;26:1095-1105.

[58] Mattson SN, Goodman AM, Caine C, Delis DC, Riley EP. Executive functioning in children with heavy prenatal alcohol exposure. *Alcohol Clin Exp Res* 1999;23:1808-1815.

[59] Wecker NS, Kramer JH, Wisniewski A, Delis DC, Kaplan E. Age effects on executive ability. *Neuropsychology* 2000;14:409-414.

[60] Beck AT, Ward CH, Mendelson M, Mock J, Erbaugh J. An inventory for measuring depression. *Arch Gen Psychiatry* 1961;4:561-571.

[61] Beck AT, Epstein N, Brown G, Steer RA. An inventory for measuring clinical anxiety: psychometric properties. *J Consult Clin Psychol* 1988;56:893-897.

[62] Krupp LB, LaRocca NG, Muir-Nash J, Steinberg AD. The fatigue severity scale. Application to patients with multiple sclerosis and systemic lupus erythematosus. *Arch Neurol* 1989;46:1121-1123.

[63] Aubry M, Cantu R, Dvorak J, et al. Summary and agreement statement of the First International Conference on Concussion in Sport, Vienna 2001. Recommendations for the improvement of safety and health of athletes who may suffer concussive injuries. *Br J Sports Med* 2002;36:6-10.

[64] Barth JT, Macciocchi SN, Giordani B, Rimel R, Jane JA, Boll TJ. Neuropsychological sequelae of minor head injury. *Neurosurgery* 1983;13:529-533.

[65] Bohnen N, Jolles J. Neurobehavioral aspects of postconcussive symptoms after mild head injury. *J Nerv Ment Dis* 1992;180:683-692.

[66] Chen JK, Johnston KM, Collie A, McCrory P, Ptito A. A validation of the post concussion symptom scale in the assessment of complex

concussion using cognitive testing and functional MRI. *J Neurol Neurosurg Psychiatry* 2007;78:1231-1238.

[67] Zhou Y, Kierans A, Kenul D, et al. Mild traumatic brain injury: longitudinal regional brain volume changes. *Radiology* 2013; 267:880-890.

[68] Colorado RA, Shukla K, Zhou Y, Wolinsky JS, Narayana PA. Multi-task functional MRI in multiple sclerosis patients without clinical disability. *Neuroimage*; 59:573-581.

[69] Mesulam M. Brain, mind, and the evolution of connectivity. *Brain Cogn* 2000;42:4-6.

[70] Bartzokis G, Lu PH, Heydari P, et al. Multimodal magnetic resonance imaging assessment of white matter aging trajectories over the lifespan of healthy individuals. *Biol Psychiatry* 2012;72:1026-1034.

[71] Bajo R, Maestu F, Nevado A, et al. Functional connectivity in mild cognitive impairment during a memory task: implications for the disconnection hypothesis. *J Alzheimers Dis* 2010;22:183-193.

[72] Zhou Y, Dougherty JH, Jr., Hubner KF, Bai B, Cannon RL, Hutson RK. Abnormal connectivity in the posterior cingulate and hippocampus in early Alzheimer's disease and mild cognitive impairment. *Alzheimers Dement* 2008;4:265-270.

[73] Glasser MF, Goyal MS, Preuss TM, Raichle ME, Van Essen DC. Trends and properties of human cerebral cortex: correlations with cortical myelin content. *Neuroimage* 2014;93 Pt 2:165-175.

[74] Ling H, Hardy J, Zetterberg H. Neurological consequences of traumatic brain injuries in sports. *Mol Cell Neurosci* 2015;66:114-122.

[75] Osborne-Crowley K, Wilson E, De Blasio F, Wearne T, Rushby J, McDonald S. Subjective emotional experience and physiological responsivity to posed emotions in people with traumatic brain injury. *Neuropsychology* 2019.

[76] Shultz SR, McDonald SJ, Corrigan F, et al. The Clinical Relevance of Behavior Testing in Animal Models of Traumatic Brain Injury. *J Neurotrauma* 2019.

[77] Covey TJ, Shucard JL, Shucard DW. Event-related brain potential indices of cognitive function and brain resource reallocation during working memory in patients with Multiple Sclerosis. *Clin Neurophysiol* 2017;128:604-621.

[78] Creed JA, DiLeonardi AM, Fox DP, Tessler AR, Raghupathi R. Concussive brain trauma in the mouse results in acute cognitive deficits and sustained impairment of axonal function. *J Neurotrauma* 2011;28:547-563.

[79] Feys P, Moumdjian L, Van Halewyck F, et al. Effects of an individual 12-week community-located "start-to-run" program on physical capacity, walking, fatigue, cognitive function, brain volumes, and structures in persons with multiple sclerosis. *Mult Scler* 2019;25:92-103.

[80] Seo JH, Park HS, Park SS, Kim CJ, Kim DH, Kim TW. Physical exercise ameliorates psychiatric disorders and cognitive dysfunctions by hippocampal mitochondrial function and neuroplasticity in post-traumatic stress disorder. *Exp Neurol* 2019;322:113043.

[81] Chen K, Fan Y, Hu R, Yang T, Li K. Impact of depression, fatigue and disability on quality of life in Chinese patients with multiple sclerosis. *Stress Health* 2013;29:108-112.

[82] Goksel Karatepe A, Kaya T, Gunaydn R, Demirhan A, Ce P, Gedizlioglu M. Quality of life in patients with multiple sclerosis: the impact of depression, fatigue, and disability. *Int J Rehabil Res* 2011;34:290-298.

[83] Zhou F, Zhuang Y, Gong H, Zhan J, Grossman M, Wang Z. Resting State Brain Entropy Alterations in Relapsing Remitting Multiple Sclerosis. *PLoS One* 2016;11:e0146080.

[84] Lepage C, de Pierrefeu A, Koerte IK, et al. White matter abnormalities in mild traumatic brain injury with and without post-traumatic stress disorder: a subject-specific diffusion tensor imaging study. *Brain Imaging Behav* 2018;12:870-881.

[85] Ren J, Lei D, Yang T, et al. Increased interhemispheric resting-state functional connectivity in paroxysmal kinesigenic dyskinesia: a resting-state fMRI study. *J Neurol Sci* 2015;351:93-98.

[86] Eskreis-Winkler S, Deh K, Gupta A, et al. Multiple sclerosis lesion geometry in quantitative susceptibility mapping (QSM) and phase imaging. *J Magn Reson Imaging* 2015;42:224-229.

[87] Wang Y, Zhong S, Jia Y, et al. Interhemispheric resting state functional connectivity abnormalities in unipolar depression and bipolar depression. *Bipolar Disord* 2015;17:486-495.

[88] Yang H, Wang C, Ji G, et al. Aberrant interhemispheric functional connectivity in first-episode, drug-naive major depressive disorder. *Brain Imaging Behav* 2019;13:1302-1310.

[89] Zhou F, Zhao Y, Huang M, Zeng X, Wang B, Gong H. Disrupted interhemispheric functional connectivity in chronic insomnia disorder: a resting-state fMRI study. *Neuropsychiatr Dis Treat* 2018;14:1229-1240.

[90] Zhou G, Liu P, Zeng F, et al. Increased interhemispheric resting-state functional connectivity in functional dyspepsia: a pilot study. *NMR Biomed* 2013;26:410-415.

[91] Li J, Gao L, Xie K, et al. Detection of Functional Homotopy in Traumatic Axonal Injury. *Eur Radiol* 2017;27:325-335.

[92] Tan X, Zhou Z, Gao J, et al. Structural connectome alterations in patients with disorders of consciousness revealed by 7-tesla magnetic resonance imaging. *Neuroimage Clin* 2019;22:101702.

[93] Wang R, Lin P, Liu M, Wu Y, Zhou T, Zhou C. Hierarchical Connectome Modes and Critical State Jointly Maximize Human Brain Functional Diversity. *Phys Rev Lett* 2019;123:038301.

[94] Zhan L, Liu Y, Wang Y, et al. Boosting brain connectome classification accuracy in Alzheimer's disease using higher-order singular value decomposition. *Front Neurosci* 2015;9:257.

[95] Vos de Wael R, Lariviere S, Caldairou B, et al. Anatomical and microstructural determinants of hippocampal subfield functional connectome embedding. *Proc Natl Acad Sci U S A* 2018;115:10154-10159.

[96] Dierks T, Frolich L, Ihl R, Maurer K. Correlation between cognitive brain function and electrical brain activity in dementia of Alzheimer type. *J Neural Transm Gen Sect* 1995;99:55-62.

[97] Helekar SA, Shin JC, Mattson BJ, et al. Functional brain network changes associated with maintenance of cognitive function in multiple sclerosis. *Front Hum Neurosci* 2010;4:219.

[98] Veltmeyer MD, Clark CR, McFarlane AC, Felmingham KL, Bryant RA, Gordon E. Integrative assessment of brain and cognitive function in post-traumatic stress disorder. *J Integr Neurosci* 2005;4:145-159.

[99] Bush G, Whalen PJ, Rosen BR, Jenike MA, McInerney SC, Rauch SL. The Counting Stroop: An interference task specialized for functional neuroimaging—Validation study with functional MRI. *Hum Brain Mapp* 1998;6:270-282.

Chapter 4

ABNORMAL MICROSTRUCTURAL CONNECTIVITY AND MORPHOMETRY IN MILD TRAUMATIC BRAIN INJURY, POST-TRAUMATIC STRESS DISORDER, MILD COGNITIVE IMPAIRMENT AND MULTIPLE SCLEROSIS

ABSTRACT

Previous studies had shown some preliminary results of white matter integrity deterioration and structural connectivity abnormalities in mild cognitive impairment (MCI), multiple sclerosis (MS), post traumatic stress disorder (PTSD) and mild traumatic brain injury (MTBI). In addition to identifying the functional network differences of the neurodegenerative diseases, the purposes of this study are to: i. investigate the microstructural DTI imaging and other morphological brain changes including volumetry under disease conditions; and ii. explore the graph-theory based small-worldness (SMW) differences in patients compared to controls of the four neurodegenerative diseases.

Microstructural FA metric identified disease-specific alterations in patients, including uncinate, major forceps, corticospinal and cingulum tracts deterioration in PTSD; significant fornix and hippocampal cingulum FA reduction in MCI; diffuse axonal injury in the frontal and occipital cortices and corpus callosum in MTBI; and lower FA in the corpus callosum and optic radiation in MS patients. In line with the abnormal micro-structure, molecular and functional imaging results, significant reductions of cortical thickness, surface area and volume involved in memory and executive function were found in PTSD and MCI patients, such as the pars opercularis, anterior cingulate, temporal pole and transverse temporal region in patients compared to controls. And finally the integrated small-worldness analyses showed similar characteristics in PTSD and AD/MCI patients, including local efficiency and small-worldness decreases but global efficiency increases. Despite no significant SMW differences in MS patients compared to controls, higher local efficiency but lower global efficiency in MTBI patients was identified additionally.

INTRODUCTION

Regarding the MRI diffusion tensor imaging (DTI) findings, significant worsening of white matter integrity had been reported in post traumatic stress disorder (PTSD) patients at different age range with various phases and causes [1, 2]. For instance, lower fractional anisotropy (FA) in the corpus callosum as well as association with anger symptoms had been found in the adolescents due to childhood abuse [3, 4]. In another study, abnormal FA in brain regions around the default-mode network and the salience network were found in children with PTSD after earthquake [5, 6]. For children with PTSD and adult-onset PTSD with childhood trauma, FA reduction in the corpus collosum was observed; however in adulthood with traumatic experience, FA changes of the cingulum, superior longitudinal fasciculus and frontal regions were reported [7-9]. Different myelin maturation age for each brain region had been reported; for instance, earlier for major forceps and thalamic radiation but latest for corticospinal tract and hippocampal cingulum [10]. In the acute phases, in a large drug-naive population who survived a specific and severe traumatic event including a major 8.0-magnitude earthquake, PTSD patients showed higher FA in the left dorsolateral prefrontal cortex white matter and forceps major, possibly related to these regional roles of fear extinction and emotion regulation [11-13].

Furthermore, in the comorbid cases, traumatic brain injury (TBI) patients with PTSD symptoms showed reduced white matter integrity in the right cingulum bundle based on axial diffusivity [14]. The comorbid mild TBI (MTBI) +PTSD group also had more abnormally lower FA clusters relative to both the healthy controls and the MTBI group without PTSD [12, 15]. In addition, significant correlations between FA and PTSD symptom severity, depression, post-concussion symptoms, reduced information processing speed had been reported [16, 17]. And strong associations were found between PTSD symptoms severity, memory accuracy, reaction time and the corpus callosum (CC) FA value in the PTSD group [18]. In addition, caudate DTI FA reductions in PTSD group but not the TBI group compared to Veteran controls were identified [19]. In MTBI with higher levels of PTSD symptom severity, loss of consciousness [20] was associated with reduced FA in the left retrolenticular part of the internal capsule [21, 22]. Compared with trauma-exposed controls, patients with PTSD showed significantly higher mean diffusivity in the right uncinate fasciculus, the major white matter tract connecting the amygdala to the prefrontal cortex [23, 24]. Furthermore, in agreement with the functional deficits in PTSD, the mean diffusivity of the right uncinate fasciculus was correlated with the fMRI activation (happy vs. neutral faces task) in the amygdala and ventromedial prefrontal cortex (vmPFC) as well as the anxiety symptoms; and FAs in the prefrontal cortex and cingulum were associated with depression and other symptoms in patients [14, 15, 25-29].

Previous studies had shown some preliminary results of white matter integrity deterioration and structural connectivity abnormalities in PTSD and TBI, mild cognitive impairment (MCI), multiple sclerosis (MS) [30-36]. In addition to identifying the functional network differences of the neurodegenerative diseases as in previous chapters, the purposes of this chapter are to: i. investigate the microstructural DTI imaging and other morphological brain changes including volumetry under disease conditions; and ii. explore the graph-theory based small-worldness (SMW) [37] differences in patients compared to controls of the four diseases.

METHODS

Participants

For microstructural DTI data analysis, FA images form the same subjects population as in chapter 2, and morphometry data from processed MRI structural T1-based Magnetization-prepared rapid acquisition gradient-echo (MPRAGE) images were downloaded from the ADNI website (www.ida.loni.usc.edu).

Methods: FA-TBSS, Morphometry and Small-Worldness Computation

Voxel-wise tract-based spatial statistics (TBSS) in FMRIB Software Library (FSL, www.fmrib.ox.ac.uk/fsl) was used to analyze DTI FA images. The MPRAGE images in each subject were processed with the Freesurfer (http://surfer.nmr.mgh.harvard.edu/) software to generate multiple brain regional cortical thickness, surface area and volume metrics for multiple dimensional territory, size and shape (1D-3D) morphological quantifications [38, 39].

SMW differences including absolute and relative, local and global efficiency parameters were quantified based on either fMRI data or cortical thickness with the algorithms outlined in our previous work [40]. For fMRI functional connectivity data as detailed in previous chapters 2, based on graph-theory, the Pearson correlation between fMRI time courses of each pair of regions of interest (ROI) was computed after preprocessing. The correlation matrix was formed with 44 Brodmann areas (BA) ROIs from MRIcro standardized landmarks (www.cabiatl.com/mricro), which was then used to generate small-world graphic topology with a threshold of $P < 0.001$ (corresponding $r > 0.265$, approximate sparsity = 50%) to maintain sparseness. For cortical thickness metrics, the thickness vector of total of 148 brain regions of interest (74 ROIs on each brain hemisphere from Freesurfer standardized landmarks) was exported from Freesurfer software to derive the Pearson correlation matrix [37]. Small world properties such as absolute clustering coefficient (C_p), absolute shortest-path length [41], relative clustering coefficient (γ, local efficiency) and relative path length (λ, global efficiency) were then computed and analyzed with in-house Matlab (http://www.mathworks.com) scripts and open resource from (http://www.stanford.edu/~dgleich/programs/matlab_bgl) in each group [10, 42]. These particular graph metrics were chosen because they have been used to study a variety of clinically important neurodegenerative and psychiatric disorders affecting the central nervous system [43, 44].

RESULTS

1. Morphometry and Microstructural Connectivity

1.1. Cortical Thickness and Volumetry

Significant reductions of cortical thickness, surface area and volume in the pars opercularis, anterior cingulate, post-central, and temporal pole as well as transverse temporal regions in PTSD patients compared to controls were found (Table 1; $P \leq 0.05$).

In MTBI patients compared to controls, no significant differences of volume at initial visit (<2 month after injury); however, significant global and regional atrophies in areas of anterior cingulate as well as isthmus white matter and precuneal gray matter were found at 1-year follow-up (corrected $P < 0.01$) [10].

Table 1. Cortical thickness and volumetry differences between PTSD patients and controls (P < 0.01)

CT = cortical thickness (mm), SA = surface area (mm^2), Vol = volume (mm^3), L = left, R = right, Pct. Diff.=Percentage of Difference between patients and controls = (patient-control)/control *100%.

ROI Name	Control	Patient	Pct. Diff.	P-value
Right Paracentral CT	2.158	2.259	-4.448	0.001
Right Pars Opercularis CT	2.337	2.407	-2.899	0.020
Right Postcentral Vol	8110.000	8527.018	-4.891	0.045
Right Rostral Anterior Cingulate CT	2.762	2.863	-3.509	0.049
Right Temporal Pole SA	433.821	461.737	-6.046	0.017
Left Accumbens Area Vol	590.571	543.164	8.728	0.043
Third Ventricle Vol	1489.964	1802.240	-17.327	0.013
Left Caudal Anterior Cingulate CT	2.383	2.585	-7.831	0.008
Left Frontal Pole CT	2.663	2.545	4.622	0.035
Left Inferior Lateral Ventricle Vol	542.714	765.538	-29.107	0.039
Left Isthmus Cingulate Vol	2835.679	2607.784	8.739	0.007
Left Isthmus Cingulate CT	2.543	2.440	4.237	0.047
Left Lateral Ventricle Vol	13887.071	18172.205	-23.581	0.028
Left Paracentral CT	2.212	2.298	-3.707	0.005
Left Pars Opercularis Vol	4112.000	4441.801	-7.425	0.036
Left Pars Opercularis SA	1497.500	1632.602	-8.275	0.016
Left Transverse Temporal Vol	1007.964	1093.556	-7.827	0.031
Left Transverse Temporal CT	2.053	2.165	-5.167	0.005

In the MCI patients, compared to controls, there was a gradual decrease of cortical thickness from MCI stables (all MMSE score ≥28) to MCI converters (at least one MMSE score < 24) [45]. The most significant thinning areas comparing MCI converters to controls were in the posterior cingulate and inferior temporal cortex with $P \leq 0.0001$. The significant cortical thinning areas ($P < 0.05$) in MCI converters compared to MCI stables were found in the regions of inferior temporal gyrus, middle frontal, posterior cingulate, pericallosal, left lateral temporo-occipital fusiform, and posterior collateral transverse temporal sulci, with the most significant reduction in the inferior temporal cortex ($P < 0.01$). The significant cortical thinning areas ($P < 0.05$) in MCI stables compared to controls were found in the inferior temporal and anterior cingulate regions.

In MS patients, using voxel-based morphometry (VBM), significantly lower brain parenchymal fraction; regional gray matter atrophy in the posterior cingulate, inferior parietal, medial prefrontal, thalamus, basal forebrain, and primary somatosensory cortex were found compared to controls ($P < 0.05$) [46].

1.2. DTI FA and TBSS Findings

20 track-based ROI quantification found lower FA in PTSD compared with control groups in the forceps major and left corticospinal tracts; with slightly higher FA in the right thalamic radiation and left uncinate fasciculus ($P = 0.05$; Table 2).

Based on voxel-wise TBSS analysis, PTSD patients had lower FA in the major forceps, thalamic radiation, cingulum, right uncinate fasciculus, corticospinal tract, superior longitudinal fasciculus and other long-distance tracts; but higher FA in the cerebellum, inferior longitudinal fasciculus, inferior fronto-occipital fasciculus as well as small temporal and occipital regions compared to controls (Figure 1, $P < 0.01$). The lower FA regions such as corticospinal tracts, cingulum and corpus callosum in PTSD can be further visualized with FSL post-processing including smoothing and bundling in Figure 2.

Significant reductions of DTI FA in MCI patients compared to controls were observed (Figure 3), especially in the tracts that connect the hippocampus such as bilateral fornix and left cingulum (Table 3, $P < 0.001$). Increment of diffusivities (both axial and radial as well as mean diffusivities) in the internal and external capsules, corpus callosum, cingulum, fornix, sagittal stratum, inferior fronto-occipital fasciculus, uncinate and superior longitudinal fasciculus in MCI patients had been observed additionally ($P < 0.001$).

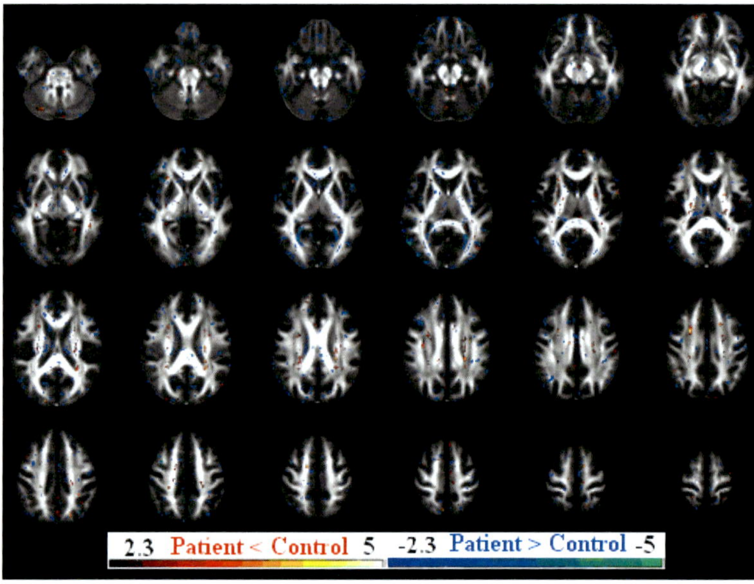

Figure 1. Based on normalized FA values, PTSD patients had lower FA (red color) in the major forceps, thalamic radiation, cingulum, right uncinate fasciculus, corticospinal tract, superior longitudinal fasciculus and other long-distance tracts including internal capsule; but higher FA in the inferior longitudinal fasciculus, inferior fronto-occipital fasciculus as well as some temporal and occipital regions in comparison to controls ($P < 0.01$).

Table 2. Track-based ROI quantification showed slight differences of FA values between PTSD and control groups in multiple brain regions, including the right thalamic radiation and left uncinate fasciculus (P = 0.05)

ROI Name	Control	Patient	Pct. Diff.	P-value
Left Anterior thalamic radiation	0.3023	0.3099	2.5158	0.1619
Right Anterior thalamic radiation	0.2977	0.3082	3.4939	0.0544
Left Corticospinal tract	0.3754	0.3678	-2.0329	0.1334
Forceps major	0.3784	0.3715	-1.8041	0.0618
Left Inferior fronto-occipital fasciculus	0.3003	0.3039	1.1712	0.0973
Left Inferior longitudinal fasciculus	0.3016	0.3037	0.7137	0.1404
Right Inferior longitudinal fasciculus	0.2334	0.2371	1.5867	0.1748
Left Uncinate fasciculus	0.2482	0.2522	1.6287	0.0513

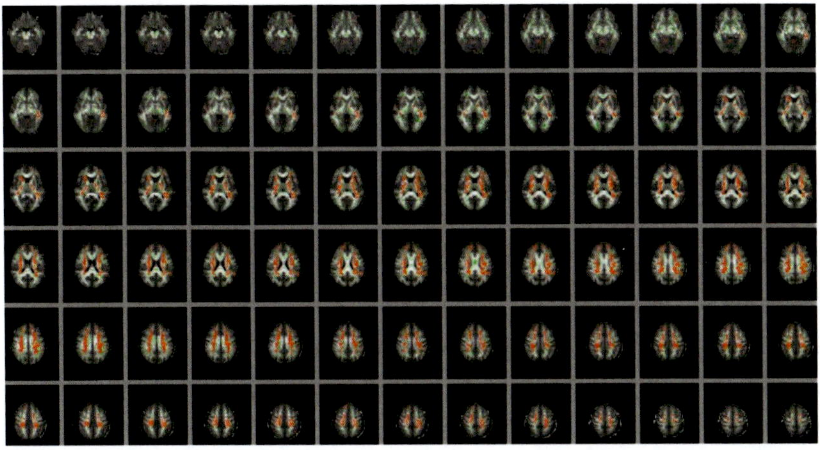

Figure 2. Lower FA (red color) in PTSD compared to controls from TBSS results (uncorrected P < 0.01) in Figure 1, processing with FSL "tbss_fill" strategy with sphere-filled smoothing kernel bundling and morphological post-processing, superimposed on white matter skeleton (green color).

Table 3. FA reduction in MCI patients compared to controls (P < 0.001)

ROI Name	Control	MCI	% Diff.	P-value
Left Cingulum (hippocampus)	0.3647	0.3580	-1.85	< 0.0001
Left Fornix (Stria terminalis)	0.3823	0.3651	-4.51	< 0.0001
Left Sagittal Stratum	0.3317	0.3190	-3.83	0.0003
Left Fornix	0.3300	0.3136	-4.97	0.0001
Right Fornix	0.4452	0.4162	-6.49	< 0.0001
Bilateral Fornix	0.4542	0.4209	-7.34	< 0.0001

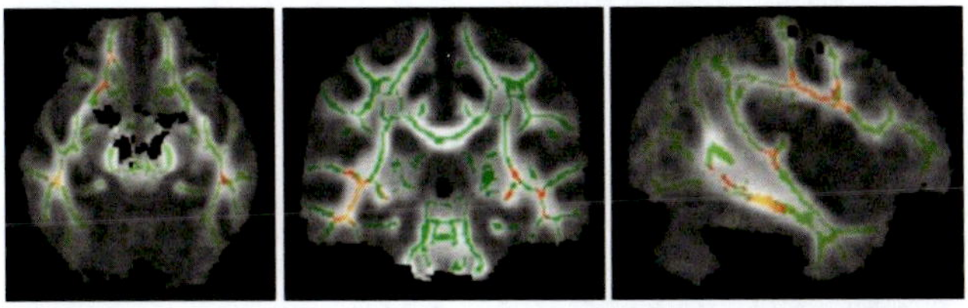

Figure 3. Lower FA (red color) in MCI compared to controls from TBSS results (whole brain threshold with FA > 0.15, and statistical comparison with P < 0.01) in regions of sagittal stratum, cingulum and superior longitudinal fasciculus. Green color indicates white matter skeleton, and small dark regions in the midbrain and superior frontal cortex that had lower FA (<0.15) was possibly due to white matter degeneration at aging.

In MTBI patients compared to controls, significant whole-brain FA reductions ($P < 0.05$), namely diffuse axonal injury (DAI), were found based on TBSS analysis and mainly in the frontal, occipital and corpus callosum areas (Figure 4) [10, 40]. In MS patients, group analysis of voxel-wise lesion probability with a threshold of probability > 0.12 (at least two subjects overlap) at baseline was shown in Figure 5a. The lesion probability map (LPM) demonstrated likely white matter (WM) lesion pattern in the periventricular regions including the frontal pole and triangle regions; with the highest probability near the top and posterior horn of the lateral ventricle. WM TBSS-based analysis showed FA reductions in MS compared to controls, predominantly in the corpus callosum, peri-ventricular areas, cingulate bundles, optic radiation and short U-fibers ($P < 0.01$) (Figure 5b). As a threshold of FA > 0.2 was applied in TBSS analysis to confine the analysis to WM, it is possible that some chronic hypointense (fluid-like) lesions were excluded. Nevertheless, the FA values of lesions were still significantly lower compared to normal appearing WM (NAWM) and lowest among all regions [46].

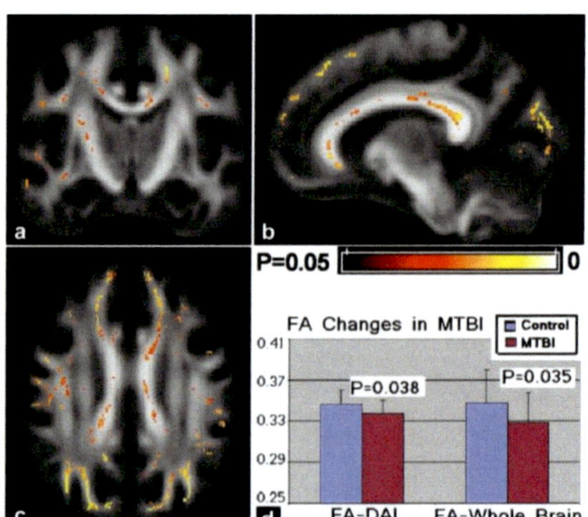

Figure 4. Whole-brain FA reductions, or diffuse axonal injury in MTBI patients compared with controls based on TBSS analysis ($P < 0.05$), mainly in the frontal, occipital and corpus callosum areas. A: Coronal view. B: Sagittal view. C: Axial views. D: Globally, MTBI patients showed reduced FA-DAI ($P = 0.038$) and FA-whole brain ($P = 0.035$) compared with controls [10, 40].

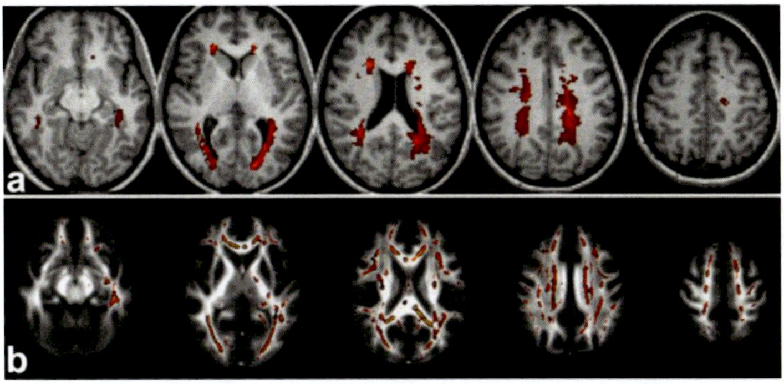

Figure 5. Representative axial slices indicated cross-sectional white matter changes in MS patients compared to controls. a: Lesion probability map (LPM) from the group analysis of voxel-wise lesion pattern with a threshold of probability >0.12, indicating the overlap lesion pattern from a minimum of two subjects. Typical WM lesion pattern was identified in the periventricular regions including the frontal pole and triangle regions. b: TBSS-based FA analysis showed FA reductions in MS patients compared to controls, predominantly in corpus callosum, periventricular areas, cingulate bundles, optic radiation and short U-fibers ($P < 0.01$) [46].

1.3. White Matter Hyperintensity Differences

There was no significant difference of whole brain WM hyperintensity lesion volume between PTSD patients and controls ($P>0.05$). In MCI cohort, a varying degree of periventricular and frontal WM lesions in both MCI patients and controls were identified, mostly due to the aging effects. Quantitative whole brain WM lesion volume was significantly higher ($P=0.002$) in MCI patients (12.88±7.47 mL) compared to controls (5.15±2.41 mL) [1]. In MS patients, typical WM lesion pattern was found in the periventricular regions including the frontal pole and triangle regions, as shown in Figure 5a.

2. Significant Graph-Theory Based SMW Differences

Table 4. SMW differences comparing PTSD to controls

Parameter	γ	λ	rel. γ	rel. λ	σ
Control	3.68	1.21	0.53	2.45	2.98
PTSD	3.05	1.18	0.48	2.54	2.56
P-value	0.0007	0.0176	0.0092	0.1124	0.0026

Both relative (rel.) and absolute local efficiency (γ) decrement (P = 0.0007 and P = 0.009, respectively; Table 4) as well as small-worldness and relative shortest path length (λ) reduction (P = 0.003 and P = 0.02 respectively) were found, indicating local efficiency reduction was accompanied with global efficiency increment in PTSD patients. In contrast to the relative global efficiency increment, the absolute global efficiency was only slightly reduced in patients, but no significant difference of SMW scale factor (σ) (P = 0.11) in PTSD..

Compared with controls, MTBI patients had lower relative betweenness centrality (measuring of global efficiency, P = 0.01), but significantly higher clustering coefficient (measuring of local efficiency, P = 0.04) [10, 40]. Furthermore, these two efficiency metrics correlated negatively with each other in patients (r = -0.77; P < 0.001). Regions with lower betweenness centrality (e.g., frontal and occipital) corresponded with the regions of reduced FA in patients, while global FA reduction correlated with betweenness centrality (r = 0.48; P = 0.03) and clustering coefficient (r = -0.46; P = 0.04) in MTBI patients. In addition, there was significantly higher thalamo-cortical connectivity that correlated with clustering coefficient (r = 0.39; P = 0.03) in patients. Also, patients with higher clustering coefficient tended to have less post concussion syndrome score with negative correlation (r = -0.4; P = 0.04).

Finally, there were significantly decreased local efficiencies in patients with MCI and AD compared to controls (P < 0.01); and MCI patients showed increased global efficiency compared to AD and controls based on the cortical thickness data [37]. The MCI converters experience the worst local efficiency during the converting period to AD; the stables, however, have highest local and global efficiency metrics. However, no significant SMW difference was found between MS patients and controls based on the previous fMRI data (P>0.05),

Discussion

Consistent with previous findings, PTSD patients showed lower FA in the right uncinate fasciculus, thalamic radiation, major forceps of the corpus callosum, cingulum, corticospinal tract and superior longitudinal fasciculus based on TBSS and track-based ROI quantification. Higher FAs in the cerebellum, left uncinate fasciculus, inferior longitudinal fasciculus, inferior fronto-occipital fasciculus as well as some temporal and occipital regions were found in PTSD patients additionally. Significantly lower FA in the corticospinal tract in PTSD patients in this relatively elderly population might also indicate age-related demyelination vulnerability of corticospinal tract given its late maturation age compared to other brain tracts and possible diffuse axonal injury after trauma [47, 48]. Reduced WM integrities in limbic-thalamo cortical tracts were implicated in combat veterans with PTSD in previous studies [26, 28]. It had also been reported that PTSD subjects had FA reduction in white matter regions of the prefrontal lobe and the posterior angular gyrus [6, 14, 15]. And similarly lower FA in the cingulum, major forceps and corticospinal tract were observed in our study, that might be due to the stress-related changes in the brain such as distraction and memory problems [49]. Higher cerebellar FA in PTSD patients might serve as a compensation role, while higher FA in the inferior longitudinal and fronto-occipital fasciculus might be related to the anxiety and hypervigilance symptom in patients [50].

Furthermore, in MCI patients compared to age-matched controls, DTI data presented significantly white matter integrity deterioration including lower FA and higher diffusivity ($P < 0.001$ and most $P < 0.0001$), most significantly in fornix and hippocampal cingulum. These regions have important memory-related links [51, 52]. MTBI patients showed globally FA reduction and diffuse axonal injury compared with controls, including the frontal and occipital regions, and the corpus callosum. MS patients showed lower FA in the corpus callosum, peri-ventricular areas, cingulate bundles, optic radiation and short U-fibers compared to controls, and lowest FA in the lesions [13, 21, 53, 54]. Consistent with previous reports [12, 50, 55, 56], different microstructural abnormalities were involved in these four diseases including largely FA reduction of hippocampal tracts in MCI, diffuse axonal injuries in MTBI, corpus callosum and optic radiation tract degeneration in MS, and corticospinal/cingulum tracts disconnectivites in PTSD patients.

In line with the abnormal frontal and temporal microstructural and functional imaging results, significant reductions of cortical thickness, surface area and volume in the pars opercularis, anterior cingulate, postcentral, and temporal pole as well as transverse temporal region in PTSD patients compared to controls based on morphometry were found in our data. Some previous work of ours [10, 45, 46] included: cortical thinning in the temporal and cingulate regions in MCI stables and converters; significant longitudinal global and regional atrophies in areas of anterior cingulate and isthmus white matter and precuneal gray matter at 1-year follow-up in MTBI; significant global and regional gray matter atrophies in the posterior cingulate, inferior parietal, medial prefrontal, thalamus, basal forebrain, and primary somatosensory cortex in MS. All the morphometry results indicated that temporal cortex and posterior cingulate cortex seem to be the typical regions involved in brain atrophy and cortical thinning in the neurodegenerative diseases.

Similar small-worldness characteristics exhibited in PTSD and MCI patients, including local efficiency and small-worldness decreases but global efficiency increases. In contrast, higher local efficiency but lower global efficiency was found in MTBI patients, with no significant SMW differences in MS patients compared with controls. Furthermore, significant functional small-world properties changes were anti-correlated in MTBI, suggesting decreased global efficiency, possibly due to diffuse axonal injury in these regions, was compensated with local network upregulation including thalamo-cortical hyper-connectivity. And abnormal cortical thickness-based small-world properties in MCI patients as well as the distinct patterns between two MCI subtypes indicated that small-world network analysis had the potential to better differentiate different stages of early dementia.

Our results of abnormal integrated brain network efficiencies based on either cortical thickness or fMRI data and regional atrophies at multiple dimensions were consistent with recently published connectome results based on structural or functional connectivities [57-60]. In addition to the main results of structural disconnectivities in these neurodegenerative diseases found in our study, some future work including correlation with other biomarkers, application to more samples at different disease stages and validation with more metrics including myelin contents are expected [61-65].

CONCLUSION

In summary, microstructural FA metric identified disease-specific white matter degeneration and alterations in patients, including uncinate, major forceps, corticospinal and cingulum tract deterioration in PTSD; significant FA reduction in the fornix and hippocampal cingulum in MCI; diffuse axonal injury in the frontal, occipital and corpus callosum in MTBI; and lastly lower FA in the corpus callosum and optic radiation in MS patients. In line with the abnormal microstructural and functional imaging results, significant reductions of cortical thickness, surface area and volume in multiple regions including temporal cortex and cingulate involved in memory and executive functions were found in all patients. And finally the integrated small-worldness analyses showed different characteristics in four diseases, including local efficiency and small-worldness decreases but global efficiency increases in PTSD and MCI, higher local efficiency but lower global efficiency in MTBI patients, and no significant differences in MS. Our results in this chapter indicated that multiple structural metrics including microstructural deterioration and morphological atrophy as well as integrated network inefficiencies reflecting neuronal resource re-routing and redistribution, demyelination, axonal injury, functional and structural disconnectivity could be used to differentiate each type of the neurodegenerative disease.

REFERENCES

[1] Bush G, Whalen PJ, Rosen BR, Jenike MA, McInerney SC, Rauch SL. The Counting Stroop: An interference task specialized for functional neuroimaging—Validation study with functional MRI. *Hum Brain Mapp* 1998;6:270-282.

[2] Dean KR, Hammamieh R, Mellon SH, et al. Multi-omic biomarker identification and validation for diagnosing warzone-related post-traumatic stress disorder. *Mol Psychiatry* 2019.

[3] Rinne-Albers MA, van der Werff SJ, van Hoof MJ, et al. Abnormalities of white matter integrity in the corpus callosum of adolescents with PTSD after childhood sexual abuse: a DTI study. *Eur Child Adolesc Psychiatry* 2016;25:869-878.

[4] Choi J, Jeong B, Polcari A, Rohan ML, Teicher MH. Reduced fractional anisotropy in the visual limbic pathway of young adults witnessing domestic violence in childhood. *Neuroimage* 2012; 59:1071-1079.

[5] Lui S, Zhou XJ, Sweeney JA, Gong Q. Psychoradiology: The Frontier of Neuroimaging in Psychiatry. *Radiology* 2016;281:357-372.

[6] Yeh PH, Wang B, Oakes TR, et al. Postconcussional disorder and PTSD symptoms of military-related traumatic brain injury associated with compromised neurocircuitry. *Hum Brain Mapp* 2014;35:2652-2673.

[7] Daniels JK, Lamke JP, Gaebler M, Walter H, Scheel M. White matter integrity and its relationship to PTSD and childhood trauma--a systematic review and meta-analysis. *Depress Anxiety* 2013; 30:207-216.

[8] Lei D, Li L, Li L, et al. Microstructural abnormalities in children with post-traumatic stress disorder: a diffusion tensor imaging study at 3.0T. Sci Rep 2015;5:8933.

[9] Siehl S, King JA, Burgess N, Flor H, Nees F. Structural white matter changes in adults and children with posttraumatic stress disorder: A

systematic review and meta-analysis. *Neuroimage Clin* 2018;19:581-598.

[10] Zhou Y. *Neuroimaging in Mild Traumatic Brain Injury.* Nova Science Publishers 2017.

[11] Clouston SAP, Deri Y, Diminich E, et al. Posttraumatic stress disorder and total amyloid burden and amyloid-beta 42/40 ratios in plasma: Results from a pilot study of World Trade Center responders. *Alzheimers Dement (Amst)* 2019;11:216-220.

[12] Lepage C, de Pierrefeu A, Koerte IK, et al. White matter abnormalities in mild traumatic brain injury with and without post-traumatic stress disorder: a subject-specific diffusion tensor imaging study. *Brain Imaging Behav* 2018;12:870-881.

[13] Li L, Lei D, Li L, et al. White Matter Abnormalities in Post-traumatic Stress Disorder Following a Specific Traumatic Event. *EBioMedicine* 2016;4:176-183.

[14] Fani N, King TZ, Jovanovic T, et al. White matter integrity in highly traumatized adults with and without post-traumatic stress disorder. *Neuropsychopharmacology* 2012;37:2740-2746.

[15] Sorg SF, Delano-Wood L, Luc N, et al. White matter integrity in veterans with mild traumatic brain injury: associations with executive function and loss of consciousness. *J Head Trauma Rehabil* 2014;29:21-32.

[16] King N. Permanent post concussion symptoms after mild head injury: a systematic review of age and gender factors. *NeuroRehabilitation* 2014;34:741-748.

[17] King NS, Kirwilliam S. Permanent post-concussion symptoms after mild head injury. *Brain Inj* 2011;25:462-470.

[18] Saar-Ashkenazy R, Veksler R, Guez J, et al. Breakdown of Inter-Hemispheric Connectivity Is Associated with Posttraumatic Symptomatology and Memory Impairment. *PLoS One* 2016;11: e0144766.

[19] Waltzman D, Soman S, Hantke NC, et al. Altered Microstructural Caudate Integrity in Posttraumatic Stress Disorder but Not Traumatic Brain Injury. *PLoS One* 2017;12:e0170564.

[20] Hillary FG, Slocomb J, Hills EC, et al. Changes in resting connectivity during recovery from severe traumatic brain injury. *Int J Psychophysiol* 2011.

[21] Hayes JP, Miller DR, Lafleche G, Salat DH, Verfaellie M. The nature of white matter abnormalities in blast-related mild traumatic brain injury. *Neuroimage Clin* 2015;8:148-156.

[22] Bolzenius JD, Velez CS, Lewis JD, et al. Diffusion Imaging Findings in US Service Members With Mild Traumatic Brain Injury and Posttraumatic Stress Disorder. *J Head Trauma Rehabil* 2018;33:393-402.

[23] Trotter BB, Robinson ME, Milberg WP, McGlinchey RE, Salat DH. Military blast exposure, ageing and white matter integrity. *Brain* 2015;138:2278-2292.

[24] Koch SBJ, van Zuiden M, Nawijn L, Frijling JL, Veltman DJ, Olff M. Decreased uncinate fasciculus tract integrity in male and female patients with PTSD: a diffusion tensor imaging study. *J Psychiatry Neurosci* 2017;42:331-342.

[25] Seminotti B, Amaral AU, Ribeiro RT, et al. Oxidative Stress, Disrupted Energy Metabolism, and Altered Signaling Pathways in Glutaryl-CoA Dehydrogenase Knockout Mice: Potential Implications of Quinolinic Acid Toxicity in the Neuropathology of Glutaric Acidemia Type I. *Mol Neurobiol* 2016;53:6459-6475.

[26] Kennis M, van Rooij SJ, Tromp do PM, et al. Treatment Outcome-Related White Matter Differences in Veterans with Posttraumatic Stress Disorder. *Neuropsychopharmacology* 2015;40:2434-2442.

[27] Lopez KC, Leary JB, Pham DL, Chou YY, Dsurney J, Chan L. Brain Volume, Connectivity, and Neuropsychological Performance in Mild Traumatic Brain Injury: The Impact of Post-Traumatic Stress Disorder Symptoms. *J Neurotrauma* 2017;34:16-22.

[28] Sanjuan PM, Thoma R, Claus ED, Mays N, Caprihan A. Reduced white matter integrity in the cingulum and anterior corona radiata in posttraumatic stress disorder in male combat veterans: a diffusion tensor imaging study. *Psychiatry Res* 2013;214:260-268.

[29] Schuff N, Zhang Y, Zhan W, et al. Patterns of altered cortical perfusion and diminished subcortical integrity in posttraumatic stress disorder: an MRI study. *Neuroimage* 2011;54 Suppl 1:S62-68.

[30] McDonald S, Dalton KI, Rushby JA, Landin-Romero R. Loss of white matter connections after severe traumatic brain injury (TBI) and its relationship to social cognition. *Brain Imaging Behav* 2019;13:819-829.

[31] McDonald WS, Jones EE, Wojciak JM, Drake RR, Sabbadini RA, Harris NG. Matrix-Assisted Laser Desorption Ionization Mapping of Lysophosphatidic Acid Changes after Traumatic Brain Injury and the Relationship to Cellular Pathology. *Am J Pathol* 2018;188:1779-1793.

[32] Shultz SR, McDonald SJ, Corrigan F, et al. The Clinical Relevance of Behavior Testing in Animal Models of Traumatic Brain Injury. *J Neurotrauma* 2019.

[33] Silver JM, McAllister TW, Yudofsky SC. *Textbook of Traumatic Brain Injury.* American Psychiatric Publishing, Inc. 2011;2nd Edition.

[34] Smith DH, Meaney DF, Shull WH. Diffuse axonal injury in head trauma. *J Head Trauma Rehabil* 2003;18:307-316.

[35] Trapp BD, Ransohoff R, Rudick R. Axonal pathology in multiple sclerosis: relationship to neurologic disability. *Curr Opin Neurol* 1999;12:295-302.

[36] Weiner MW, Harvey D, Hayes J, et al. Effects of traumatic brain injury and posttraumatic stress disorder on development of Alzheimer's disease in Vietnam Veterans using the Alzheimer's Disease Neuroimaging Initiative: Preliminary Report. *Alzheimers Dement* (N Y) 2017;3:177-188.

[37] Zhou Y, Lui YW. Small-World Properties in Mild Cognitive Impairment and Early Alzheimer's Disease: A Cortical Thickness MRI Study. *ISRN Geriatr* 2013;542080.

[38] Fischl B, Salat DH, van der Kouwe AJ, et al. Sequence-independent segmentation of magnetic resonance images. *Neuroimage* 2004;23 Suppl 1:S69-84.

[39] Fischl B. FreeSurfer. *Neuroimage* 2012;62:774-781.

[40] Zhou Y. Small world properties changes in mild traumatic brain injury. *J Magn Reson Imaging* 2017;46:518-527.

[41] Briggs DI, Defensor E, Memar Ardestani P, et al. Role of Endoplasmic Reticulum Stress in Learning and Memory Impairment and Alzheimer's Disease-Like Neuropathology in the PS19 and APP(Swe) Mouse Models of Tauopathy and Amyloidosis. *eNeuro* 2017;4.

[42] Zhou Y. Functional Neuroimaging Methods and Frontiers. *Nova Science Publishers.* 2018.

[43] Dickerson BC, Bakkour A, Salat DH, et al. The cortical signature of Alzheimer's disease: regionally specific cortical thinning relates to symptom severity in very mild to mild AD dementia and is detectable in asymptomatic amyloid-positive individuals. *Cereb Cortex* 2009;19:497-510.

[44] He Y, Chen Z, Evans A. Structural insights into aberrant topological patterns of large-scale cortical networks in Alzheimer's disease. *J Neurosci* 2008;28:4756-4766.

[45] Zhou Y. *Functional Neuroimaging with Multiple Modalities: Principles, Devices and Applications*. Nova Science Publishers 2016.

[46] Zhou Y. *Neuroimaging in Multiple Sclerosis.* Nova Science Publishers 2017.

[47] Bartzokis G, Lu PH, Heydari P, et al. Multimodal magnetic resonance imaging assessment of white matter aging trajectories over the lifespan of healthy individuals. *Biol Psychiatry* 2012;72:1026-1034.

[48] Bourbon-Teles J, Bells S, Jones DK, Coulthard E, Rosser A, Metzler-Baddeley C. Myelin Breakdown in Human Huntington's Disease: Multi-Modal Evidence from Diffusion MRI and Quantitative Magnetization Transfer. *Neuroscience* 2019;403:79-92.

[49] Hoffman AN, Taylor AN. Stress reactivity after traumatic brain injury: implications for comorbid post-traumatic stress disorder. *Behav Pharmacol* 2019;30:115-121.

[50] Matthews SC, Spadoni AD, Lohr JB, Strigo IA, Simmons AN. Diffusion tensor imaging evidence of white matter disruption associated with loss versus alteration of consciousness in warfighters exposed to combat in Operations Enduring and Iraqi Freedom. *Psychiatry Res* 2012;204:149-154.

[51] Alosco ML, Sugarman MA, Besser LM, et al. A Clinicopathological Investigation of White Matter Hyperintensities and Alzheimer's Disease Neuropathology. *J Alzheimers Dis* 2018;63:1347-1360.

[52] Boespflug EL, Storrs J, Sadat-Hossieny S, et al. Full diffusion characterization implicates regionally disparate neuropathology in mild cognitive impairment. *Brain Struct Funct* 2014;219:367-379.

[53] Matthews PM, Roncaroli F, Waldman A, et al. A practical review of the neuropathology and neuroimaging of multiple sclerosis. *Pract Neurol* 2016;16:279-287.

[54] Ukueberuwa DM, Arnett PA. Coping style as a protective factor for emotional consequences of structural neuropathology in multiple sclerosis. *J Clin Exp Neuropsychol* 2019;41:390-398.

[55] Klimova A, Korgaonkar MS, Whitford T, Bryant RA. Diffusion Tensor Imaging Analysis of Mild Traumatic Brain Injury and Posttraumatic Stress Disorder. *Biol Psychiatry Cogn Neurosci Neuroimaging* 2019;4:81-90.

[56] Kontos AP, Van Cott AC, Roberts J, et al. Clinical and Magnetic Resonance Spectroscopic Imaging Findings in Veterans With Blast Mild Traumatic Brain Injury and Post-Traumatic Stress Disorder. *Mil Med* 2017;182:99-104.

[57] Wang J, Khosrowabadi R, Ng KK, et al. Alterations in Brain Network Topology and Structural-Functional Connectome Coupling Relate to Cognitive Impairment. *Front Aging Neurosci* 2018;10:404.

[58] Xiao F, Lei D, An D, et al. Functional brain connectome and sensorimotor networks in rolandic epilepsy. *Epilepsy Res* 2015;113:113-125.

[59] Zhou Y. *Traumatic Brain Injury: Neurbiology, Diagnosis and Treatment.* Editor, Intechopen Publisher 2019.

[60] Zhou J, Gennatas ED, Kramer JH, Miller BL, Seeley WW. Predicting regional neurodegeneration from the healthy brain functional connectome. *Neuron* 2012;73:1216-1227.

[61] Adnan A, Crawley A, Mikulis D, Moscovitch M, Colella B, Green R. Moderate-severe traumatic brain injury causes delayed loss of white matter integrity: evidence of fornix deterioration in the chronic stage of injury. *Brain Inj* 2013;27:1415-1422.

[62] Bierer LM, Ivanov I, Carpenter DM, et al. White matter abnormalities in Gulf War veterans with posttraumatic stress disorder: A pilot study. *Psychoneuroendocrinology* 2015;51:567-576.

[63] Feeney C, Sharp DJ, Hellyer PJ, et al. Serum insulin-like growth factor-I levels are associated with improved white matter recovery after traumatic brain injury. *Ann Neurol* 2017;82:30-43.

[64] Peters JM, Struyven RR, Prohl AK, et al. White matter mean diffusivity correlates with myelination in tuberous sclerosis complex. *Ann Clin Transl Neurol* 2019;6:1178-1190.

[65] Bartzokis G, Lu PH, Mintz J. Human brain myelination and amyloid beta deposition in Alzheimer's disease. *Alzheimers Dement* 2007;3:122-125.

Chapter 5

ABNORMAL MOLECULAR IMAGING INCLUDING TAU, AMYLOID AND FDG IN MILD TRAUMATIC BRAIN INJURY, POST-TRAUMATIC STRESS DISORDER, MILD COGNITIVE IMPAIRMENT AND MULTIPLE SCLEROSIS

ABSTRACT

Some preliminary results of tau and amyloid imaging as well as neuroinflammation and metabolism dysfunction in various neurodegenerative diseases including PTSD, MTBI and MCI had been reported recently. In addition to identifying the functional and structural network differences of the neurodegenerative diseases, the purpose of this chapter is to quantify further available molecular imaging tracers such as tau, amyloid and FDG-glucose in the four neurodegenerative diseases.

The results demonstrated significantly different molecular imaging biomarkers patterns for distinguishing each neurodegenerative. . In PTSD patients compared to controls, both regional quantification and Braak staging algorithm found significantly higher tau in the temporal, parietal and visual cortices such as hippocampus, anterior and posterior cingulate, precuneus and planum polare regions at stages II and later Braak stages VI, V and IV. While in MCI patients compared to controls, higher tau deposition was found in the early possible pathological regions of entorhinal, hippocampal and temporal cortices with significantly higher tau only in the early Braak stages I and II. Higher tau in the typical vmPFC and temporal region in PTSD patients in contrast to the higher tau in the thalamic/hypothalamic and orbitofrontal regions in TBI indicated different but overlapped neuropathological burdens of these two diseases. PTSD patients also had significantly higher amyloid accumulation in the temporal, occipital and inferior parietal lobes; while MCI patients showed higher degree of amyloid depositions both globally and regionally in the medial prefrontal and posterior cingulate cortices compared to controls. Different patterns of tau and amyloid depositions in MCI patients compared to PTSD/TBI and controls were exhibited, including higher tau at early Braak stages in MCI vs. much higher tau at later Braak stages in PTSD and higher at subcortical regions in TBI. Hypometabolism of glucose based on FDG PET imaging in PTSD and MCI patients compared to controls had been observed additionally. Our advanced neuroimaging quantifications including multiple molecular tracers demonstrated significant and distinct brain alterations at various scales in different types of neurodegenerative diseases with high sensitivity and specificity.

INTRODUCTION

Both amyloid and tau deposition are the neuropathological hallmarks of neurodegenerative diseases [1]. These two most widely studied imaging tracers have been applied to Alzheimer's disease (AD) and associated with memory and cognitive dysfunction [2-6]. At which stages are they involved in other neurodegenerative diseases such as chronic stress disorder in PTSD and TBI patients, and how they relate to disease recovery need to be further investigated [7-9]. Reports related to molecular imaging including tau and amyloid applications in PTSD were relatively limited, with a couple of recent findings [10, 11].

One study had found widespread tau accumulation in neocortical regions in PTSD and TBI groups, with no significant differences of tau distribution between PTSD and comorbid PTSD+TBI group [12]. Also the extent of tauopathy was positively correlated with the neuropsychological deficit scores such as Alzheimer's disease assessment scale (ADAS) in PTSD patients. TBI patients had shown widely scattered tau tangles in the frontal and posterior parietal/temporal regions based on neuropathological examination [13]. Higher accumulations of amyloid in the frontal, occipital and temporal lobes of PTSD that suffers with significant cognitive dysfunction compared to controls had been reported, as well as higher amyloid in the white matter of comorbid PTSD+TBI group. In addition, the correlations between amyloid PET results and CSF markers of neuropathology in the TBI and PTSD+TBI groups had been confirmed [14].

Some hypotheses of amyloidosis and tauopathy in PTSD and TBI have been proposed recently [1, 12, 15-17]. For instance, stress-related metabolic changes including hypothalamic-pituitary-adrenal (HPA) axis dysfunction [18], hippocampal atrophy and aberrant connections between hypothalamus and hippocampus had been observed in the previous chapters. Higher metabolic stress in some brain regions including medial prefrontal cortex (MPFC) and posterior cingulate cortex (PCC) may be more vulnerable to amyloid neurotoxicity and might lead to further amyloid aggregation at early disease stage [19-22]. Furthermore, in the trauma cases, when the severe mechanical stress arises rapidly, the tau-crosslinked microtubules integrity might breakdown and cause tau dissociation and aggregation [23-27]. Especially in the gray matter-white matter junctions, the axonal cytoskeleton damage due to the shearing forces after trauma and the abnormal tau nucleation could promote abnormal neurofibrillation tangle (NFT) formation, leading to tauopathy in PTSD and TBI [14, 28, 29]. Several PET tracers for labeling demyelination, myelin repair, immune system activation and neurodegeneration in multiple sclerosis (MS) have been developed recently [30].

For instance, the peripheral benzodiazepine receptor, specifically the translocator protein (TSPO) [(11)]C-PK11195 PET tracer targeting neuroinflammation had shown higher uptake in the white matter lesions and was correlated with clinical disability [31]. Additionally, TSPO-[(18)F]DPA-714 PET tracer had higher uptake in the gray matter regions such as hippocampus and thalamus for labeling neurodegeneration in MS disease model [32].

Previous studies had shown some preliminary results of tau and amyloid imaging as well as neuroinflammation and metabolism dysfunction in various neurodegenerative diseases including PTSD, TBI, MS and AD including mild cognitive impairment (MCI) [14, 26, 30-35]. In addition to identifying the functional and structural network differences of the neurodegenerative diseases, the purpose of this chapter is to quantify further available molecular imaging tracers such as tau accumulation, amyloid deposition and Fluoro-2-deoxyglucose (FDG)-glucose metabolism in the four neurodegenerative diseases.

METHODS

Participants

For the same participants in previous chapters, multiparametric imaging data including molecular tracers of amyloid, tau and FDG-glucose images at multiple visits, and processed regional quantifications including volumetry were downloaded from the ADNI website (www.ida.loni. usc.edu).

ROI-Quantification, FA-TBSS, Voxel-Wise Normalization and Comparison

Both [^{18}-F] AV-1451 (for tau tangle labeling) and [^{18}-F] AV-45 (for amyloid plaque), as well as [^{18}-F] FDG (for glucose metabolism) PET images were analyzed to derive the ratio of standard uptake value (SUVR) choosing cerebellum as the tissue reference with in-house developed scripts. Namely, after normalization to the standard Montreal Neurologic Institute (MNI) space with the FMRIB, Software Library (FSL, http://fsl.fmrib.ox.ac.uk/fsl), a well-validated atlas of total 116 regions of interest covering whole brain cortical and subcortical areas was used as regional parcellation. Braak stage ROIs were derived from the atlas definitions by Scholl et al. [36, 37]. Statistical comparisons between patients and controls of imaging metrics such as tau deposition, amyloid accumulation and FDG uptake were implemented using FSL and MATLAB software (www.mathematics.com).

RESULTS

1. Molecular Imaging in PTSD and TBI Patients

1.1. Tau Imaging

Control subject demonstrated relatively low tau deposition across the brain, except a few non-specific binding regions such as in the subcortical thalamus (Figure 1a). In contrast, for the PTSD patient, much higher tau deposition was found in the vmPFC and inferior temporal regions primarily (Figure 1b).

However, for the TBI patient, higher tau deposition was found in the thalamus, hypothalamus and orbitofrontal regions. These regions were more vulnerable to injury in TBI patients (Figure 2a). As expected, for another PTSD patient, higher tau deposition was found consistently in the vmPFC and inferior temporal regions (Figure 2b) compared to other brain regions.

Group-wise tau quantification revealed typical lower tau deposition pattern in control group (mean of all six Braak stages ≤1.2 SUVR) (Figure 3), highest in Stage II and much lower in other stages. Compared to controls, significantly higher tau deposition in PTSD patients especially at later Braak stages regions such as stage VI ($P = 0.005$), V ($P = 0.016$) and

IV (P = 0.029) as well as typical tau deposition in Braak stage II (P = 0.013) were observed with mean tau ≥1.2 for stages II to VI.

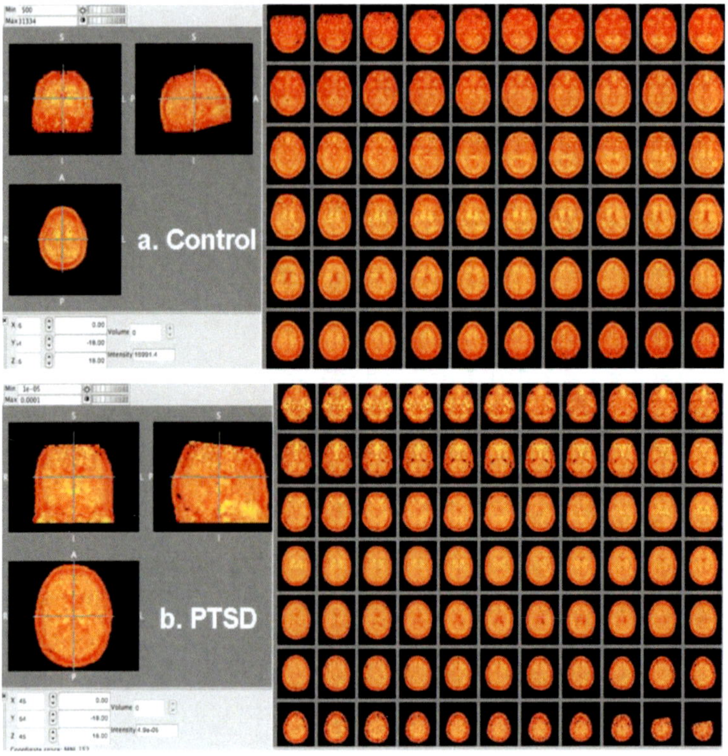

Figure 1a. Control participant: relatively low tau deposition across the brain; b. PTSD patient: higher tau deposition was found in the vmPFC and inferior temporal regions.

Furthermore, whole brain voxel-based statistical comparison results revealed significantly higher tau depositions ($P<0.01$) in the areas of vmPFC, somatosensory, superior temporal, cingulate, precuneus, lingual, parietal and motor areas in PTSD patients compared to controls; with lower tau deposition in areas of cerebellum, occipital and some temporal regions in patients (Figure 4). Consistent with voxel-wise results, ROI-based quantification presented higher tau depositions in PTSD patients at the regions of bilateral cingulate, precuneus, lingual, parietal perculum, as well as left hippocampus and thalamus, left putamen, right intracalcarine cortex and right planum polare (Table 1).

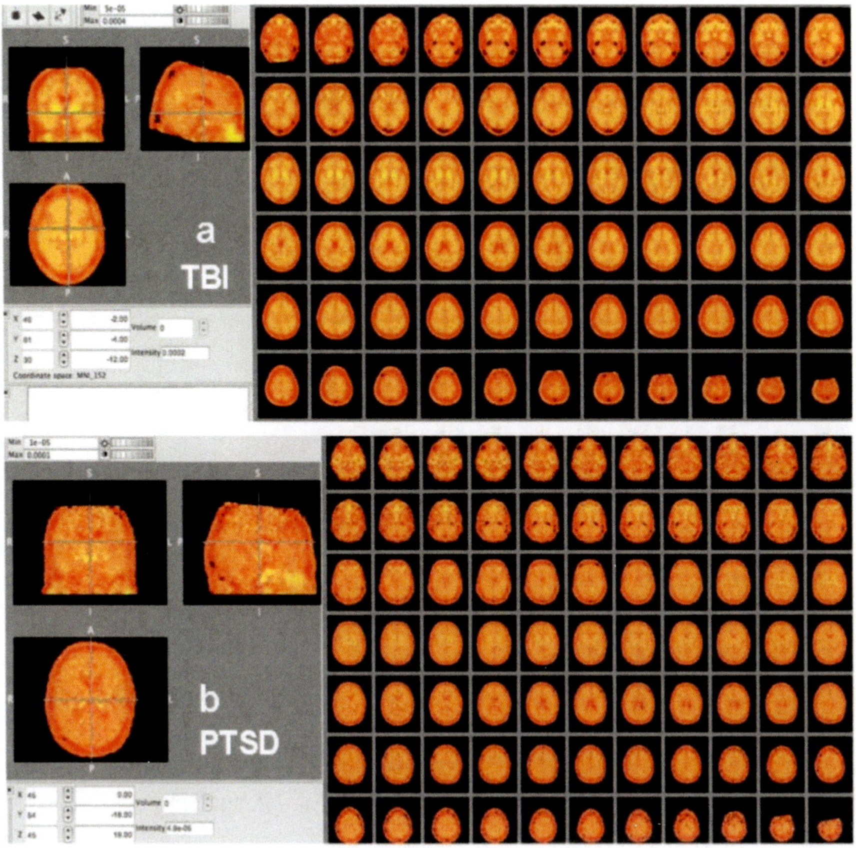

Figure 2a. TBI patient: higher tau deposition was found in the thalamus, hypothalamus and orbitofrontal regions; b. Another representative PTSD patient: typical pattern of higher tau deposition in the vmPFC and inferior temporal regions.

Specifically, 116-regional ROI-based quantification showed higher tau depositions ($P < 0.01$) in PTSD patients compared to controls, at Braak stage II-VI areas including the regions of left hippocampus (stage II); left lingual gyrus (stage III); bilateral anterior and posterior cingulate (stage IV), left thalamus (stage IV); bilateral precuneus (stage V), left putamen (stage V), left parietal operculum (stage V), right planum polare (stage V); right intracalcarine cortex (stage VI) (Table 1; $P < 0.01$). Lower tau in the right lingual gyrus and parietal operculum cortex were found additionally.

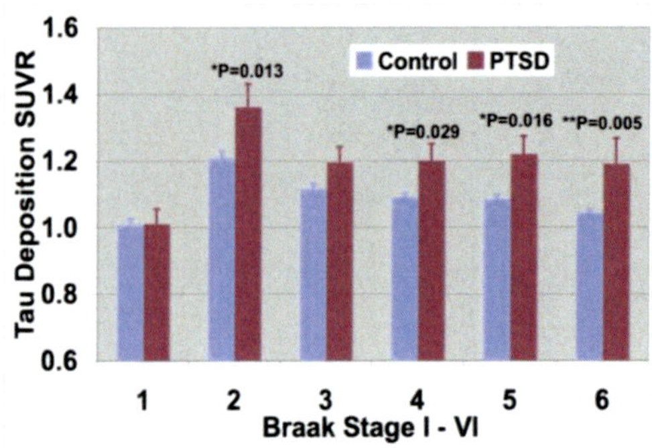

* marked significant difference with P < 0.05; and ** for P < 0.01.

Braak stage I:	entorhinal cortex.
Braak stage II:	hippocampus.
Braak stage III:	amygdala, parahippocampus, lingual, and fusiform gyri.
Braak stage IV:	inferior temporal cortex; middle temporal cortex; temporal pole, thalamus, insula; the caudal, rostral, isthmus and posterior of cingulate.
Braak stage V:	frontal cortex; parietal cortex; occipital cortex; transverse, superior temporal cortex; precuneus; banks of superior temporal sulcus; nucleus accumbens; caudate nucleus; putamen.
Braak stage VI:	precentral gyrus; postcentral gyrus; paracentral gyrus; cuneus; pericalcarine.

Figure 3. Significantly higher tau deposition in PTSD patients compared to controls; especially at later Braak stages such as stage VI (P = 0.005), V (P = 0.16) and IV (P = 0.029) as well as typical tau deposition regions in Braak stage II (P = 0.013). And the Braak stage area definition was based on the previously published atlas [36].

Table 1. Significant ROI-based tau differences between PTSD and controls with Braak staging (P < 0.01)

ROI Name	Control	Patient	Pct Diff.	P-value
L Cingulate Gyrus, anterior division (IV)	0.8947	0.9676	8.1500	0.0017
L Cingulate Gyrus, posterior division (IV)	1.0831	1.1325	4.5606	0.0035
L Precuneus Cortex (V)	0.8742	0.9995	14.3265	0.0094
L Lingual Gyrus (III)	0.9622	1.0530	9.4362	0.0031
L Parietal Operculum Cortex (V)	1.0047	1.0658	6.0851	0.0058
L Thalamus (IV)	1.0152	1.0857	6.9459	0.0053
L Putamen (V)	0.9535	1.1034	15.7239	0.0097
L Hippocampus (II)	1.1551	1.2142	5.1181	0.0057
R Intracalcarine Cortex (VI)	1.1265	1.2437	10.4018	0.0083
R Cingulate Gyrus, anterior division (IV)	1.0881	1.1109	2.0999	0.0072
R Cingulate Gyrus, posterior division (IV)	1.1309	1.1979	5.9311	0.0070
R Precuneus Cortex (V)	1.1053	1.1859	7.2893	0.0053
R Lingual Gyrus	1.0887	1.0542	-3.1715	0.0086
R Parietal Operculum Cortex	1.1531	0.9080	-21.2590	0.0074
R Planum Polare	0.9762	1.0472	7.2793	0.0088

* Pct. Diff. (Percent Difference, %.) = (Patient-Control)/Control*100; L = Left, R = Right.

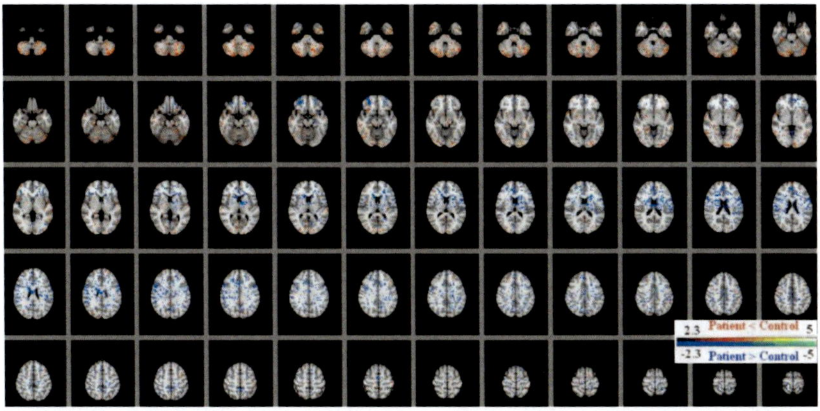

Figure 4. Whole brain voxel-based results showed higher tau depositions in areas of vmPFC, posterior cingulate, somatosensory, superior temporal, parietal, precuneus, lingual and motor areas were observed in PTSD patients (blue color) ($P < 0.01$); however, cerebellum, occipital and some temporal regions had lower tau SUVR (red color) in patients compared to controls.

1.2. Amyloid Imaging

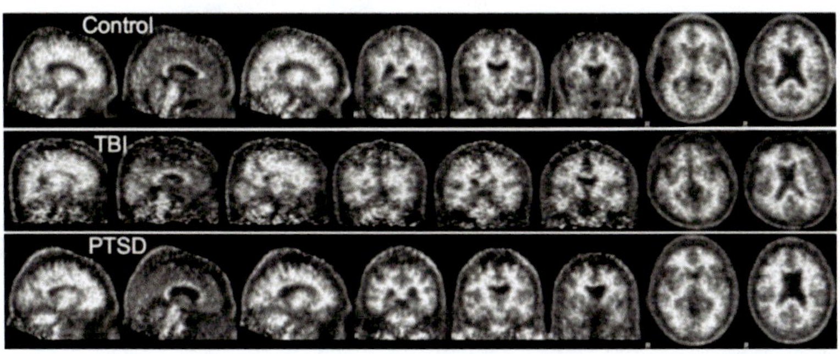

Figure 5. Representation images of amyloid deposition in TBI and PTSD patients compared to controls; showing relatively higher amyloid in the parietal, occipital and frontal regions in PTSD patient and possibly higher amyloid uptake in the subcortical areas in TBI patient.

Regarding amyloid plaques, higher amyloid accumulation in the temporal, occipital and inferior parietal lobe were observed in PTSD patients based on voxel-wise comparison results (Figures 5 and 6), with lower amyloid in small regions of the medial prefrontal, superior parietal, posterior cingulate and cuneus ($P < 0.01$). Based on ROI analysis, significantly higher Aβ in the pallidum and brainstem but lower in the superior parietal lobe in PTSD patients were found, compared to controls ($P < 0.01$; Table 2).

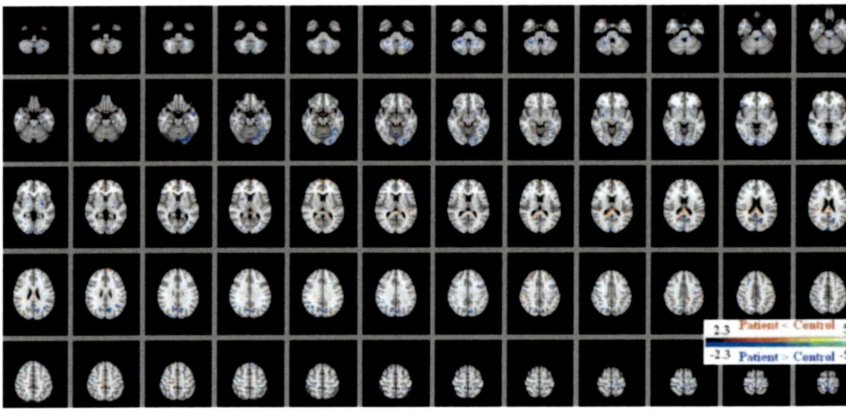

Figure 6. Higher amyloid accumulations in scattered regions in the inferior portion of the vmPFC, temporal, occipital and superior parietal lobes were observed in PTSD patients (blue color) ($P < 0.01$), with lower amyloid in small regions of the medial prefrontal, posterior cingulate, motor and cuneus (red color).

Table 2. Significant ROI-based Aβ differences between PTSD and controls ($P < 0.01$)

ROI Name	Control	Patient	Pct. Diff.	P-value
L Superior Parietal Lobule	0.9662	0.9607	-0.5688	0.0350
L Pallidum	1.0706	1.1007	2.8106	0.0310
L Brainstem	0.9056	0.9913	9.4578	0.0364

Molecular imaging data of MCI patients had been reported in our previous work at both baseline and longitudinal visits [1, 37]. For the tau deposition comparison, significantly higher ($P < 0.05$) tau accumulations in MCI patients compared to controls were found in regions of hippocampus, temporal fusiform, frontal operculum cortex, cuneus, and accumbens based on ADNI data. Furthermore, significant correlations between tau accumulations in the temporal cortex including fusiform, inferior as well as middle segments and composite memory score in MCI patients were found ($P<0.01$) [38]. For the amyloid deposition, global cerebral cortex amyloid uptake (i.e., SUVR) showed a higher-degree of amyloid deposition in patients with MCI (1.42 ± 0.15) compared with controls (1.15 ± 0.12), both with $P < 0.001$ [38]. Regional SUVR quantification also demonstrated significantly higher uptake values in MCI patients compared to controls ($P < 0.001$), including the posterior cingulate cortex (PCC) ($P < 0.005$; SUVR of 1.56 ± 0.33 in MCI vs. 1.15 ± 0.21 in controls) and medial prefrontal cortex (MPFC) ($P < 0.005$; 1.66 ± 0.35 in MCI vs. 1.20 ± 0.35 in controls).

1.3. FDG Imaging

Table 3. Significant correlations between initial volumetry and follow-up FDG uptake in MCI group (P < 0.01)

ROI Name	Correlation	P-value
Left Entorhinal Volume and mean Posterior Cingulate FDG	-0.3316	0.0079
Left Entorhinal Volume and median Posterior Cingulate FDG	-0.3272	0.0089
Left Entorhinal Volume and maximal Posterior Cingulate FDG	-0.3233	0.0097
Left Inferior Parietal Volume and mode Angular FDG	-0.3224	0.0100
Right Inferior Parietal Volume and median Angular FDG	-0.3554	0.0043
Left Entorhinal Volume and mode Right Temporal FDG	-0.3477	0.0052
Left Entorhinal Volume and minimal Right Temporal FDG	-0.3477	0.0052
Left Amygdala Volume and mode Right Temporal FDG	-0.3407	0.0063
Left Amygdala Volume and minimal Right Temporal FDG	-0.3407	0.0063
Left Inferior Parietal Volume and minimal Left Angular FDG	-0.3224	0.0100
Right Inferior Parietal Volume and minimal Angular FDG	-0.3554	0.0043

Global hypometabolism of glucose based on FDG imaging in PTSD patients compared to controls was found ($P = 0.047$, percent difference = -6.9%; global centered mean of 0.648 for PTSD vs. 0.696 for control).

For the MCI patients, there was significantly lower cerebral FDG SUVR in patients compared to controls ($P = 0.002$). Furthermore, longitudinal date indicated that significant correlations existed between the volumes of entorhinal, amygdala, inferior parietal cortex at initial visit and the FDG uptake (mean, minimal, maximal, median and mode metrics of SUVR) at 12-month follow-up in the posterior cingulate, angular and temporal cortices ($P < 0.01$). Detailed results are summarized in Table 3.

Discussion

Our results indicated significantly different molecular imaging patterns for distinguishing each neurodegenerative disease. For instance, although the chronic traumatic encephalography (CTE) might be the causes of the memory disorder in PTSD and TBI [39], the patterns of the tau distribution of PTSD and MCI were quite different. In the PTSD patients, significantly higher tau depositions were found mainly at later Braak stages (IV, V and V) in addition to the expected higher tau deposition regions in Braak stage II in the hippocampus. However, in the preclinical MCI elderly samples, higher tau depositions were found only in the early possible pathological regions of entorhinal, hippocampal and temporal cortices with highest tau at early Braak stages I and II, in agreement with previous findings [1, 36, 39, 40]. Both regional quantification and Braak staging algorithm found consistent results, including significantly higher tau in the vmPFC, temporal, parietal and visual cortices as well as as hippocampus, anterior and posterior cingulate, precuneus and planum polare regions at stages II, VI, V and IV for the PTSD patients compared to normal aging participants. These regions play important roles in memory, learning, emotional regulation, executive function, attention control, visual and auditory information processing that haven often been found deficits in stress disorder patients [11, 41-43]. On the other hand, our results also demonstrated higher tau depositions in the subcortical thalamic/hypothalamic and orbitofrontal regions in TBI in contrast to the higher tau in cortical regions including typical vmPFC and inferior temporal cortex in PTSD patients, suggesting overlapped (both involving vmPFC) but different (more subcortical thalamic and hypothalamic regions for TBI) neuropathological burdens of two diseases. In summary, different patterns of tau depositions in MCI patients compared to PTSD/TBI and controls were exhibited, suggesting high-specificity of tau tracer for distinct region-specific distributions of neuropathological burden of each disease.

Regarding the amyloid deposition, significantly higher degree of amyloid depositions were observed in MCI patients compared to controls, both globally and regionally such as in the medial prefrontal cortex and posterior cingulate, consistent with recent studies [37, 44-49]. In PTSD patients, our results showed higher amyloid accumulation in the temporal, occipital and inferior parietal lobes with slightly lower amyloid in small regions of the medial prefrontal, posterior cingulate, superior parietal and cuneus. Global hypometabolism of FDG glucose had been observed in both PTSD and MCI patients compared to controls ($P < 0.05$) additionally. Our molecular imaging results were in agreement with recently reported values in the four neurodegenerative diseases [7, 11-13, 29]. And significant correlations between the volumes of entorhinal, amygdala, inferior parietal cortex at initial visit and the follow-up FDG uptake in the posterior cingulate, angular and temporal cortices indicating the atrophy in the temporal cortex might lead to the hypometabolism of glucose in regions that have important functions of learning and memory in MCI [1, 38, 50, 51].

Although both amyloid deposition and tau accumulation were higher in PTSD/TBI/MCI patients, the specific regions involved in each disease were quite different from each other, possibly due to various disease mechanisms [43, 52-54]. In PTSD patients, it is possible that trauma events induce NFT formation around small blood vessels, and cause blood-brain barrier damage. The cerebrovascular injury will increase arterial stiffness and further facilitates amyloid and tau deposition. Both abnormal intracellular tau and extracellular amyloid, together with white matter deterioration and neuronal activity/connectivity dysfunction might be the unique biomarkers of this chronic stress-related disorder [55-60]. In the MCI patients, more extracellular amyloid deposition and intracellular tau accumulation act as trigger and bullet, to cause neuronal death in brain, especially in the specific temporal cortex starting with the entorhinal region and hippocampus [2]. Brain dysfunction in the default mode network with aging and more amyloid depositions in these regions are the typical imaging findings of MCI patients [52, 61, 62]. With the disease progresses, more amyloid deposition globally, tau spreading and hypometabolism in the posterior regions including temporal and parietal cortices are usually observed in the neurodegenerative cases [1, 37, 63].

CONCLUSION

In summary, we had reported significant differences of imaging biomarkers including molecular, functional, microstructural and morphological data for detecting neurodegenerative diseases from controls. Primary molecular results included higher tau tangles and amyloid plaques in the vmPFC and temporal regions in the PTSD and TBI patients compared to controls, as well as global glucose hypometabolism. Higher but different patterns of tau and amyloid depositions in MCI patients compared to PTSD/TBI and controls were found including higher tau at early Braak stages I and II in MCI in contrast to the higher tau accumulation at later Braak stages IV-VI in PTSD and higher at subcortical regions in TBI. Our multiple neuroimaging quantifications in this book demonstrated significant and distinct brain alterations at various scales in different types of neurodegenerative diseases with high sensitivity and specificity. These comprehensive imaging features and the illustrative applications had cross-validated each other finding, and could be integrated to provide a broad and complete disease imaging profile for the purpose of improving diagnosis accuracy and treatment efficiency.

ACKNOWLEDGMENTS

Data collection and sharing for this project was funded by the Alzheimer's Disease Neuroimaging Initiative (ADNI) (National Institutes of Health Grant U01 AG024904) and DOD ADNI (Department of Defense award number W81XWH-12-2-0012). ADNI is funded by the National Institute on Aging, the National Institute of Biomedical Imaging and Bioengineering, and through generous contributions from the following: AbbVie, Alzheimer's Association; Alzheimer's Drug Discovery Foundation; Araclon Biotech; BioClinica, Inc.; Biogen; Bristol-Myers Squibb Company; CereSpir, Inc.; Cogstate; Eisai Inc.; Elan Pharmaceuticals, Inc.; Eli Lilly and Company; EuroImmun; F. Hoffmann-

La Roche Ltd and its affiliated company Genentech, Inc.; Fujirebio; GE Healthcare; IXICO Ltd.; Janssen Alzheimer Immunotherapy Research and Development, LLC.; Johnson and Johnson Pharmaceutical Research and Development LLC.; Lumosity; Lundbeck; Merck and Co., Inc.; Meso Scale Diagnostics, LLC.; NeuroRx Research; Neurotrack Technologies; Novartis Pharmaceuticals Corporation; Pfizer Inc.; Piramal Imaging; Servier; Takeda Pharmaceutical Company; and Transition Therapeutics. The Canadian Institutes of Health Research is providing funds to support ADNI clinical sites in Canada. Private sector contributions are facilitated by the Foundation for the National Institutes of Health (www.fnih.org). The grantee organization is the Northern California Institute for Research and Education, and the study is coordinated by the Alzheimer's Therapeutic Research Institute at the University of Southern California. ADNI data are disseminated by the Laboratory for NeuroImaging at the University of Southern California.

Data used in preparation of this article were obtained from the Alzheimer's Disease Neuroimaging Initiative (ADNI) database website (adni.loni.usc.edu). The author is one of the investigators of ADNI data cohort. The other investigators within the ADNI might contribute to the design and implementation of ADNI and/or provide data but did not participate in analysis or writing of this report.

REFERENCES

[1] Zhou Y. *Function and Metabolism of Aging: Longitudinal Neuroimaging Evaluation.* Nova Science Publishers 2019.

[2] Jack CR, Jr., Knopman DS, Jagust WJ, et al. Hypothetical model of dynamic biomarkers of the Alzheimer's pathological cascade. *Lancet Neurol* 2010;9:119-128.

[3] Morris MC, Compas BE, Garber J. Relations among posttraumatic stress disorder, comorbid major depression, and HPA function: a systematic review and meta-analysis. *Clin Psychol Rev* 2012;32:301-315.

[4] Schwarz AJ, Yu P, Miller BB, et al. Regional profiles of the candidate tau PET ligand 18F-AV-1451 recapitulate key features of Braak histopathological stages. *Brain* 2016;139:1539-1550.

[5] Smith R, Puschmann A, Scholl M, et al. 18F-AV-1451 tau PET imaging correlates strongly with tau neuropathology in MAPT mutation carriers. *Brain* 2016;139:2372-2379.

[6] Yang B, Wang Z, Sheng C, et al. Evidence-based review of oral traditional Chinese medicine compound recipe administration for treating weight drop-induced experimental traumatic brain injury. *BMC Complement Altern Med* 2016;16:95.

[7] Im JJ, Namgung E, Choi Y, Kim JY, Rhie SJ, Yoon S. Molecular Neuroimaging in Posttraumatic Stress Disorder. *Exp Neurobiol* 2016;25:277-295.

[8] Erlich SS, Fleming JO, Stohlman SA, Weiner LP. Experimental neuropathology of chronic demyelination induced by a JHM virus variant (DS). *Arch Neurol* 1987;44:839-842.

[9] Yaffee HS. Trauma and pustular psoriasis. *J Am Acad Dermatol* 1985;13:1055-1057.

[10] Pattinson CL, Gill JM, Lippa SM, Brickell TA, French LM, Lange RT. Concurrent Mild Traumatic Brain Injury and Posttraumatic Stress Disorder Is Associated With Elevated Tau Concentrations in Peripheral Blood Plasma. *J Trauma Stress* 2019;32:546-554.

[11] Weiner MW, Harvey D, Hayes J, et al. Effects of traumatic brain injury and posttraumatic stress disorder on development of Alzheimer's disease in Vietnam Veterans using the Alzheimer's Disease Neuroimaging Initiative: Preliminary Report. *Alzheimers Dement* (N Y) 2017;3:177-188.

[12] Mohamed AZ, Cumming P, Srour H, et al. Amyloid pathology fingerprint differentiates post-traumatic stress disorder and traumatic brain injury. *Neuroimage Clin* 2018;19:716-726.

[13] Pattinson CL, Shahim P, Taylor P, et al. Elevated Tau in Military Personnel Relates to Chronic Symptoms Following Traumatic Brain Injury. *J Head Trauma Rehabil* 2019.

[14] Clouston SAP, Deri Y, Diminich E, et al. Posttraumatic stress disorder and total amyloid burden and amyloid-beta 42/40 ratios in plasma: Results from a pilot study of World Trade Center responders. *Alzheimers Dement (Amst)* 2019;11:216-220.

[15] Ling H, Hardy J, Zetterberg H. Neurological consequences of traumatic brain injuries in sports. *Mol Cell Neurosci* 2015;66:114-122.

[16] Shultz SR, McDonald SJ, Corrigan F, et al. The Clinical Relevance of Behavior Testing in Animal Models of Traumatic Brain Injury. *J Neurotrauma* 2019.

[17] Zetterberg H, Winblad B, Bernick C, et al. Head trauma in sports - clinical characteristics, epidemiology and biomarkers. *J Intern Med* 2019;285:624-634.

[18] Rangaprakash D, Deshpande G, Daniel TA, et al. Compromised hippocampus-striatum pathway as a potential imaging biomarker of mild-traumatic brain injury and posttraumatic stress disorder. *Hum Brain Mapp* 2017;38:2843-2864.

[19] Gardner RC, Burke JF, Nettiksimmons J, Kaup A, Barnes DE, Yaffe K. Dementia risk after traumatic brain injury vs nonbrain trauma: the role of age and severity. *JAMA Neurol* 2014;71:1490-1497.

[20] Jellinger KA. Traumatic brain injury and Alzheimer's disease neuropathology. Alzheimers Dement 2019.

[21] Schmidt U, Willmund GD, Holsboer F, et al. Searching for non-genetic molecular and imaging PTSD risk and resilience markers: Systematic review of literature and design of the German Armed Forces PTSD biomarker study. *Psychoneuroendocrinology* 2015;51:444-458.

[22] Sugarman MA, McKee AC, Stein TD, et al. Failure to detect an association between self-reported traumatic brain injury and Alzheimer's disease neuropathology and dementia. *Alzheimers Dement* 2019;15:686-698.

[23] Bandak FA, Ling G, Bandak A, De Lanerolle NC. Injury biomechanics, neuropathology, and simplified physics of explosive

blast and impact mild traumatic brain injury. *Handb Clin Neurol* 2015;127:89-104.

[24] Bigler ED. Neuropathology of Mild Traumatic Brain Injury: Correlation to Neurocognitive and Neurobehavioral Findings. In: Kobeissy FH, ed. *Brain Neurotrauma: Molecular, Neuropsychological, and Rehabilitation Aspects.* Boca Raton (FL), 2015.

[25] Bigler ED, Maxwell WL. Neuropathology of mild traumatic brain injury: relationship to neuroimaging findings. *Brain Imaging Behav* 2012;6:108-136.

[26] Fidan E, Lewis J, Kline AE, et al. Repetitive Mild Traumatic Brain Injury in the Developing Brain: Effects on Long-Term Functional Outcome and Neuropathology. *J Neurotrauma* 2016;33:641-651.

[27] Taber KH, Hurley RA. Update on mild traumatic brain injury: neuropathology and structural imaging. *J Neuropsychiatry Clin Neurosci* 2013;25:1-5.

[28] McKee AC, Robinson ME. Military-related traumatic brain injury and neurodegeneration. *Alzheimers Dement* 2014;10:S242-253.

[29] Mohamed AZ, Cumming P, Gotz J, Nasrallah F, Department of Defense Alzheimer's Disease Neuroimaging I. Tauopathy in veterans with long-term posttraumatic stress disorder and traumatic brain injury. *Eur J Nucl Med Mol Imaging* 2019;46:1139-1151.

[30] Matthews PM, Roncaroli F, Waldman A, et al. A practical review of the neuropathology and neuroimaging of multiple sclerosis. *Pract Neurol* 2016;16:279-287.

[31] Rissanen E, Tuisku J, Rokka J, et al. In Vivo Detection of Diffuse Inflammation in Secondary Progressive Multiple Sclerosis Using PET Imaging and the Radioligand [(11)]C-PK11195. *J Nucl Med* 2014;55:939-944.

[32] Zinnhardt B, Belloy M, Fricke IB, et al. Molecular Imaging of Immune Cell Dynamics During De- and Remyelination in the Cuprizone Model of Multiple Sclerosis by [(18)F]DPA-714 PET and MRI. *Theranostics* 2019;9:1523-1537.

[33] Briggs DI, Defensor E, Memar Ardestani P, et al. Role of Endoplasmic Reticulum Stress in Learning and Memory Impairment

and Alzheimer's Disease-Like Neuropathology in the PS19 and APP(Swe) Mouse Models of Tauopathy and Amyloidosis. *eNeuro* 2017;4.

[34] Yuan M, Pantazatos SP, Zhu H, et al. Altered amygdala subregion-related circuits in treatment-naive post-traumatic stress disorder comorbid with major depressive disorder. *Eur Neuropsychopharmacol* 2019.

[35] Zhou Y. *Neuroimaging in Multiple Sclerosis.* Nova Science Publishers 2017.

[36] Scholl M, Lockhart SN, Schonhaut DR, et al. PET Imaging of Tau Deposition in the Aging Human Brain. *Neuron* 2016;89:971-982.

[37] Zhou Y, Bai B. Tau and Pet/Mri Imaging Biomarkers for Detecting and Diagnosing Early Dementia. *Jacobs J Med Diagn Med Imaging* 2017;2.

[38] Zhou Y, Yu F, Duong TQ, Alzheimer's Disease Neuroimaging I. White matter lesion load is associated with resting state functional MRI activity and amyloid PET but not FDG in mild cognitive impairment and early Alzheimer's disease patients. *J Magn Reson Imaging* 2015;41:102-109.

[39] Silver JM, McAllister TW, Yudofsky SC. *Textbook of Traumatic Brain Injury.* American Psychiatric Publishing, Inc. 2011;2nd Edition.

[40] Zhao Q, Liu M, Ha L, Zhou Y, Alzheimer's Disease Neuroimaging I. Quantitative (18)F-AV1451 Brain Tau PET Imaging in Cognitively Normal Older Adults, Mild Cognitive Impairment, and Alzheimer's Disease Patients. *Front Neurol* 2019;10:486.

[41] Buckner RL, Snyder AZ, Shannon BJ, et al. Molecular, structural, and functional characterization of Alzheimer's disease: evidence for a relationship between default activity, amyloid, and memory. *J Neurosci* 2005;25:7709-7717.

[42] Raichle ME, Snyder AZ. A default mode of brain function: a brief history of an evolving idea. *Neuroimage* 2007;37:1083-1090; discussion 1097-1089.

[43] Villemagne VL, Okamura N. Tau imaging in the study of ageing, Alzheimer's disease, and other neurodegenerative conditions. *Curr Opin Neurobiol* 2016;36:43-51.

[44] Chandra A, Valkimadi PE, Pagano G, et al. Applications of amyloid, tau, and neuroinflammation PET imaging to Alzheimer's disease and mild cognitive impairment. *Hum Brain Mapp* 2019.

[45] Di Benedetto G, Burgaletto C, Carta AR, et al. Beneficial effects of curtailing immune susceptibility in an Alzheimer's disease model. *J Neuroinflammation* 2019;16:166.

[46] DeKraker J, Ferko KM, Lau JC, Kohler S, Khan AR. Unfolding the hippocampus: An intrinsic coordinate system for subfield segmentations and quantitative mapping. *Neuroimage* 2018;167:408-418.

[47] Fang XX, Sun GL, Zhou Y, Qiu YH, Peng YP. TGF-beta1 protection against Abeta1-42-induced hippocampal neuronal inflammation and apoptosis by TbetaR-I. *Neuroreport* 2018;29:141-146.

[48] Vos de Wael R, Lariviere S, Caldairou B, et al. Anatomical and microstructural determinants of hippocampal subfield functional connectome embedding. *Proc Natl Acad Sci U S A* 2018;115:10154-10159.

[49] Jiao SS, Shen LL, Zhu C, et al. Brain-derived neurotrophic factor protects against tau-related neurodegeneration of Alzheimer's disease. *Transl Psychiatry* 2016;6:e907.

[50] Francati V, Vermetten E, Bremner JD. Functional neuroimaging studies in posttraumatic stress disorder: review of current methods and findings. *Depress Anxiety* 2007;24:202-218.

[51] Hughes KC, Shin LM. Functional neuroimaging studies of post-traumatic stress disorder. *Expert Rev Neurother* 2011;11:275-285.

[52] Jack CR, Jr., Bennett DA, Blennow K, et al. A/T/N: An unbiased descriptive classification scheme for Alzheimer disease biomarkers. *Neurology* 2016;87:539-547.

[53] Jack CR, Jr., Knopman DS, Jagust WJ, et al. Tracking pathophysiological processes in Alzheimer's disease: an updated

hypothetical model of dynamic biomarkers. *Lancet Neurol* 2013;12:207-216.

[54] Ossenkoppele R, Schonhaut DR, Scholl M, et al. Tau PET patterns mirror clinical and neuroanatomical variability in Alzheimer's disease. *Brain* 2016;139:1551-1567.

[55] Alosco ML, Sugarman MA, Besser LM, et al. A Clinicopathological Investigation of White Matter Hyperintensities and Alzheimer's Disease Neuropathology. *J Alzheimers Dis* 2018;63:1347-1360.

[56] Davis PC, Gearing M, Gray L, et al. The CERAD experience, Part VIII: Neuroimaging-neuropathology correlates of temporal lobe changes in Alzheimer's disease. *Neurology* 1995;45:178-179.

[57] Hanfelt JJ, Peng L, Goldstein FC, Lah JJ. Latent classes of mild cognitive impairment are associated with clinical outcomes and neuropathology: Analysis of data from the National Alzheimer's Coordinating Center. *Neurobiol Dis* 2018;117:62-71.

[58] Murayam S, Saito Y. [Neuropathology of mild cognitive impairment Alzheimer's disease]. *Rinsho Shinkeigaku* 2007;47:912-914.

[59] Schneider JA, Arvanitakis Z, Leurgans SE, Bennett DA. The neuropathology of probable Alzheimer disease and mild cognitive impairment. *Ann Neurol* 2009;66:200-208.

[60] Sousa Alves G. CSF beta-amyloid and white matter damage: unravelling the neuropathology of Alzheimer's disease. *J Neurol Neurosurg Psychiatry* 2018;89:329.

[61] Jack CR, Jr., Wiste HJ, Weigand SD, et al. Defining imaging biomarker cut points for brain aging and Alzheimer's disease. *Alzheimers Dement* 2016.

[62] Dean KR, Hammamieh R, Mellon SH, et al. Multi-omic biomarker identification and validation for diagnosing warzone-related post-traumatic stress disorder. *Mol Psychiatry* 2019.

[63] Brier MR, Gordon B, Friedrichsen K, et al. Tau and Abeta imaging, CSF measures, and cognition in Alzheimer's disease. *Sci Transl Med* 2016;8:338ra366.

Chapter 6

MORE APPLICATIONS OF NEUROIMAGING IN THERAPEUTIC EVALUATION AND NEW HORIZON

ABSTRACT

Previous studies including ours had demonstrated many applications of fcMRI in quantifying therapeutic evidence, evaluating treatment efficacy such as traditional Chinese medicine (TCM) and implementation in other challenging diseases. The purposes of this study are to review some of the therapeutic effects of TCM with neuroimaging quantifications to help treating neurodegenerative diseases, and to summarize some imaging applications in other challenging diseases.

INTRODUCTION

Previous studies had demonstrated many applications of functional connectivity with MRI (fcMRI) in quantifying therapeutic evidence, evaluating treatment efficacy of medicine such as traditional Chinese medicine (TCM) [1-3], as well as expanding to some new horizons including mind reading [4, 5] and neuroplasticity enhancement [3, 6]. The purposes of this chapter are to: i. review some of the therapeutic effects of TCM with neuroimaging quantifications to help treating neurodegenerative diseases including post-traumatic stress disorder (PTSD), traumatic brain injury (TBI), multiple sclerosis (MS) and Alzheimer's disease (AD) with quantitative imaging evaluations; and ii. summarize the generalization of imaging techniques in evaluating associated brain changes of treatment effects for other challenging diseases including cancer.

SECTION I. TCM, MS, AD AND TBI TREATMENT

Neuroimaging provides the quantitative and scientific evaluation of therapeutic medicines with noninvasive and *in vivo* perspectives to the disease mechanism in the brain. Multiparametric imaging is of pivotal importance to reveal the complex pathophysiologies of many challenging diseases including chronic neurodegenerative diseases as discussed in previous chapters. In some life-threatening diseases such as cancer, the needs of effective treatments expand to the well-known complementary and alternative medicine (CAM) [7]. One of the most explored and famous (from about years of 800 BC) CAM is the Chinese medicine. Chinese herbal medicine (CHM) or traditional Chinese medicine (TCM) and acupuncture are the two major components of Chinese medicine, with some supplementations such as Tai Chi Chuan [8-10]. The main philosophy of TCM is to gain energy and maintain balances of body, mind and environment for a better harmonic life with thoroughly recorded and scientifically evaluated Chinese herbs [11, 12]. For treating brain disorders, as well-documented and confirmed by many recent studies [12], TCM has numerous beneficial treatment effects including neuroprotective, anti-inflammatory, anti-oxidative, nutrition and longevity functions [13-16].

MS is a chronic inflammatory demyelinating disease. During the disease course, the autoimmune inflammation process activates the macrophages to destroy myelin, that could trigger white matter deterioration, vascular inflammation and neurodegeneration [17, 18].

Disease mechanism consists mainly of energy imbalance, ion accumulation, neuroinflammation, oxidative and metabolic stress. Multiple sub-cellular molecules that mediate the disease progression of initial inflammation and later demyelination, axonal injury, metabolic dysfunction and neuronal damage include nitric oxide (NO) and reactive oxygen species (ROS) [19]. Oligodendrocyte death, demyelination, axonal damage, neuronal death, formation of glial scars, and excitotoxicity are the common manifestation of the disease that could lead to the disability in MS patients. 85% of MS patients are the relapsing-remitting (RR) MS (RRMS) with months to years of relapses; and about 55–65% of RRMS develop the secondary progressive MS (SPMS) when disease worsen and disability accumulates [20-22].

In addition to the western medicine such as rituximab, over 50% MS patients may use CAM for neuroprotection, nutrition and anti-oxidative properties [20, 23]. One of the widely used TCM, *Ginkgo biloba* tablets (GBT) can improve the therapeutic efficacy, cognitive ability, and cerebral blood flow supply of patients [24]. Studies had shown that GBT could inhibit inducible NO syntheses (iNOS) [25] expression, lead to better NO bioavailability and endothelial function, and have neuroprotective effect by preventing nerve cells from apoptosis after spinal cord injury in rats [26]. Further pharmacological studies confirmed that *Ginkgo* elicited anti-oxidant and anti-radical effects, facilitated microcirculation with higher cerebral blood flow, improved neural plasticity and memory, lowered brain injuries and the risks of possible neurodegenerative disease, as well as reduced fatigue and symptom severity [27-29].

Gastrodin, a famous Chinese herb for treating diseases for centuries, has effects on anti-oxidation, anti-inflammation and suppressing microglial activation [30]. Repeated treatment with gastrodin could reverse the enhanced single prolonged stress (ESPS)-induced PTSD symptoms including anxiety and further lower iNOS, and therefore possesses the anxiolytic effect. Both Albiflorin extracted from radix paeoniae Alba and inulin-type oligosaccharides of morinda officinalis had been effective in treating depression syndrome, with better allopregnanolone biosynthesis in the prefrontal cortex, hippocampus, and amygdala of the brain [31].

Furthermore, electroacupuncture (EA) pretreatment ameliorates ESPS-induced anxiety-like behaviors and prevents hippocampal neurogenesis disruption in a rat model of PTSD possibly through regulation of the keap1/Nrf2 antioxidant defense pathway [32, 33]. Tai Chi Chuan had improved cardiovascular function, musculoskeletal condition, and reduction of anxiety, especially in chronic conditions; as demonstrated by many recent studies [34, 35]. 6-week of Tai Chi practice in TBI patients had revealed increased happiness and energy, with significant improvements in emotion regulation including sadness, confusion, anger, tension, and fear compared to a control group. Tai chi could also help relieve the chronic distress symptoms of PTSD [34, 36].

Chinese herbal medicine, acupuncture, and Tai Chi Chuan were found to have beneficial effects in patients with TBI [35, 36]. Proving to be a clinically useful therapy for several brain disorders, acupuncture could increase the excitability of the corticospinal system; implicating that acupuncture might accelerate the recovery of motor function in patients with disorders of consciousness following TBI [37]. Gypenoside had been reported to have neuroprotective effects, regulate nerve-regulating factors, and help the proliferation of neural stem cells that could finally improve the recovery of neurological functions such as memory and learning in TBI patients [15, 38, 39]. NeuroAid, a TCM compound that contains 14 different herb components, invented and synthesized in China, had neuroprotective and neurorestorative actions in animal models and improved cognitive function following TBI [40-43].

Ethanol extract of TCM Centipeda minima [44] had been found to have the antioxidant and neuroprotective effects by alleviating oxidative stress that were implicated in the pathogenesis of neurodegeneration and other aging-related diseases [45, 46]. Scutellarin (SC), extracted from the Chinese herb *Erigeron breviscapus,* was reported to reduce the deposition of amyloid β1-42 (Aβ1-42) and the expression of phosphorylated-tau in the hippocampus. And therefore SC could provide the protective effects in dementia including mild cognitive impairment (MCI) [47]. Cistanches herba and its extracts could improve learning and memory of dementia patients and memory-deficient rats [48-51]. Rhizoma Alismatis has been shown to ameliorate memory dysfunction, and protect the ultrastructure of the cerebral cortex due to aging and therefore has been used as a therapeutic TCM for senile dementia, especially in AD [52-54]. Research on polygonum multiflorum thumb and its extracts suggested that it may have beneficial effect on hippocampal neurons through the suppression of ROS accumulation [55]. Bushen capsules (BSCs), the classic TCM formulas, had positive effects on episodic and working memory in MCI patients [56-58]. And the BSCs therapy had improved the connectivity and efficiency of resting state default mode network (DMN) [59-61].

SECTION II. NEW HORIZON INCLUDING FUNCTIONAL CONNECTIVITY APPLICATIONS IN TUMOR, CANCER AND HIV

Our previous studies indicated that functional connectivity metric generated from various brain networks had high region-seeded network specificity to detect brain circuit dysfunction in neurodegenerative diseases, and was associated with the clinical symptoms and many other imaging metrics. Some further applications of functional connectivity in other challenging diseases are reviewed in this section.

Studies on brain tumors such as glioblastoma and meningioma had demonstrated that tumors presented a remarkable different resting-state blood oxygen level-dependent (BOLD) signal when compared to surrounding tissue [62]. For example, Chow et al. showed that the temporal profile of the fMRI BOLD signal in glioblastoma exhibited some overlap with peritumoral regions [63]. The bilateral motor and sensorimotor networks in the tumor exhibited reduced connectivity compared to contralateral hemisphere. Loss of connectivity in default mode and executive control networks, and association with reduced cognitive function in cancer patients were reported recently [64]. Furthermore, fatigued breast cancer survivors had alterations in brain neurochemistry within the posterior insula and disturbed DMN functional connectivity in comparison to non-fatigued breast cancer survivors [65].

Functional connectivity can also be used to evaluate chemotherapy effects for cancer treatment. Imaging results demonstrated lower dorsal attention network functional connectivity at one month after chemotherapy, but higher at one year in patients [54, 66-69]. This observation was also consistent with the cognitive deficits in chemotherapy patients in the domains of attentional processing and executive functioning. On the other hand, DMN connectivity was decreased both at one month and one year following chemotherapy [70].

Some specific subsystems such as the lateral occipital cortex, DMN, salience network and cortico-striatal network may be altered in subjects with human immunodeficiency virus (HIV) infection that is a major challenging disease worldwide [71]. Using both advanced non-linear analysis of resting-state fMRI and graph theory, statistically significant associations of small worldness with neuropsychological testing results were found in HIV patients. Largely preserved brain function and integrity based on structural connectivity analysis during Acute HIV infection (AHI) [72] and indication for the preservation of brain integrity during chronic HIV through early and persistent viral suppression with antiretroviral treatment (ART) had been observed as well [73, 74]. AHI individuals also exhibited lower functional connectivity between the parahippocampal cortex of the DMN and the left middle frontal gyrus after ART exposure in contrast to no exposure. Combination ART (cART) [75] reduces both glial activation and inflammation caused by HIV, leading to increases in neuronal synchronous activity that is reflected within specific canonical resting state networks [76, 77]. And it had been shown that HIV+ individuals with cART had greater resting-state functional connectivity in certain networks than cART- individuals. Some TCM such as Ganoderma lucidum and red Ginseng had been effective in treating cancer and HIV diseases [78-80]. Finally, combination of TCM and the modern therapies such as highly active antiretroviral therapy (HAART) for treating difficult diseases, better quality of life and greater survival rate are expected with enhanced brain function in patients [54, 81, 82].

REFERENCES

[1] Moreno-Ortega M, Prudic J, Rowny S, et al. Resting state functional connectivity predictors of treatment response to electroconvulsive therapy in depression. *Sci Rep* 2019;9:5071.

[2] Vik BMD, Skeie GO, Vikane E, Specht K. Effects of music production on cortical plasticity within cognitive rehabilitation of patients with mild traumatic brain injury. *Brain Inj* 2018;32:634-643.

[3] Yang M, He H, Duan M, et al. The Effects of Music Intervention on Functional Connectivity Strength of the Brain in Schizophrenia. *Neural Plast* 2018;2018:2821832.

[4] Bohl V, van den Bos W. Toward an integrative account of social cognition: marrying theory of mind and interactionism to study the interplay of Type 1 and Type 2 processes. *Front Hum Neurosci* 2012;6:274.

[5] Gakis M, Cichoń E, Cyrkot T, Szczepanowski R. Consciousness and Social Cognition from an Interactionist Perspective: A New Approach on Understanding Normal and Abnormal Relations between Metacognition and Mindreading. I*ntechopen Publisher, Prefrontal Cortex* 2018.

[6] Dukic H. Music, Brain Plasticity and the Resilience: The Pillars of New Receptive Therapy. *Psychiatr Danub* 2018;30:141-147.

[7] Chow WH, Chang P, Lee SC, Wong A, Shen HM, Verkooijen HM. Complementary and alternative medicine among Singapore cancer patients. *Ann Acad Med Singapore* 2010;39:129-135.

[8] Jiang HL, Niu JJ, Zhang WF, et al. The role of central nervous system on hypoglycemia and the feasibility of the brain theory in traditional Chinese medicine on treatment of diabetes mellitus. *J Integr Med* 2014;12:1-6.

[9] May BH, Feng M, Zhou IW, et al. Memory Impairment, Dementia, and Alzheimer's Disease in Classical and Contemporary Traditional Chinese Medicine. *J Altern Complement Med* 2016;22:695-705.

[10] Zhou J, Yin T, Gao Q, Yang XC. A Meta-Analysis on the Efficacy of Tai Chi in Patients with Parkinson's Disease between 2008 and 2014. *Evid Based Complement Alternat Med* 2015;2015:593263.

[11] Yang B, Wang Z, Sheng C, et al. Evidence-based review of oral traditional Chinese medicine compound recipe administration for treating weight drop-induced experimental traumatic brain injury. *BMC Complement Altern Med* 2016;16:95.

[12] Wu D, Shen Y, Ye B, et al. Efficacy and advantages of modified Traditional Chinese Medicine treatments based on "kidney reinforcing" for chronic aplastic anemia: A randomized controlled clinical trial. *J Tradit Chin Med* 2016;36:434-443.

[13] Chen G, Lu C, Zha Q, et al. A network-based analysis of traditional Chinese medicine cold and hot patterns in rheumatoid arthritis. *Complement Ther Med* 2012;20:23-30.

[14] Chen Z, Lin SY, Zhou YH, et al. [Analysis of clinical features of traditional Chinese medicine symptoms and syndromes of 220 patients with chronic aplastic anemia]. *Zhongguo Zhong Xi Yi Jie* He Za Zhi 2014;34:43-45.

[15] Zhao CQ, Zhou Y, Ping J, Xu LM. Traditional Chinese medicine for treatment of liver diseases: progress, challenges and opportunities. *J Integr Med* 2014;12:401-408.

[16] Zhou Y. [International exchanges in the early stage of the Academy of Traditional Chinese Medicine]. *Zhonghua Yi Shi Za Zhi* 2015;45:330-332.

[17] Filippi M, Bruck W, Chard D, et al. Association between pathological and MRI findings in multiple sclerosis. *Lancet Neurol* 2019;18:198-210.

[18] Kasahata N, Murayama S, Shiota J. [A clinico-pathological study of so-called "acute multiple sclerosis" mimicking a brain tumor on the MRI findings]. *Rinsho Shinkeigaku* 1999;39:327-332.

[19] Lim YY, Hassenstab J, Cruchaga C, et al. BDNF Val66Met moderates memory impairment, hippocampal function and tau in preclinical autosomal dominant Alzheimer's disease. *Brain* 2016;139:2766-2777.

[20] Song L, Zhou QH, Wang HL, et al. Chinese herbal medicine adjunct therapy in patients with acute relapse of multiple sclerosis: A systematic review and meta-analysis. *Complement Ther Med* 2017;31:71-81.

[21] Zhou D, Srivastava R, Nessler S, et al. Identification of a pathogenic antibody response to native myelin oligodendrocyte glycoprotein in multiple sclerosis. *Proc Natl Acad Sci U S A* 2006;103:19057-19062.

[22] Zhou Y, Chen M, Simpson S, Jr., et al. Common genetic variation within miR-146a predicts disease onset and relapse in multiple sclerosis. *Neurol Sci* 2018;39:297-304.

[23] Killestein J, Rudick RA, Polman CH. Oral treatment for multiple sclerosis. *Lancet Neurol* 2011;10:1026-1034.

[24] Ao Q, Sun XH, Wang AJ, et al. Protective effects of extract of Ginkgo biloba (EGb 761) on nerve cells after spinal cord injury in rats. *Spinal Cord* 2006;44:662-667.

[25] He D, Zhou H, Guo D, Hao Z, Wu B. Pharmacologic treatment for memory disorder in multiple sclerosis. *Cochrane Database Syst Rev* 2011:CD008876.

[26] Lovera J, Bagert B, Smoot K, et al. Ginkgo biloba for the improvement of cognitive performance in multiple sclerosis: a randomized, placebo-controlled trial. *Mult Scler* 2007;13:376-385.

[27] Wang XD, Lu H, Shi Z, et al. A Pilot Study on Clinical and Neuroimaging Characteristics of Chinese Posterior Cortical Atrophy: Comparison with Typical Alzheimer's Disease. *PLoS One* 2015;10:e0134956.

[28] Yin J, Zhang H, Ye J. Traditional chinese medicine in treatment of metabolic syndrome. *Endocr Metab Immune Disord Drug Targets* 2008;8:99-111.

[29] Johnson SK, Diamond BJ, Rausch S, Kaufman M, Shiflett SC, Graves L. The effect of Ginkgo biloba on functional measures in multiple sclerosis: a pilot randomized controlled trial. *Explore* (NY) 2006;2:19-24.

[30] Liu Y, Gao J, Peng M, et al. A Review on Central Nervous System Effects of Gastrodin. *Front Pharmacol* 2018;9:24.

[31] Qiu ZK, Liu CH, Gao ZW, et al. The inulin-type oligosaccharides extract from morinda officinalis, a traditional Chinese herb, ameliorated behavioral deficits in an animal model of post-traumatic stress disorder. *Metab Brain Dis* 2016;31:1143-1149.

[32] Wang Z, Dong H, Wang Q, et al. Effects of electroacupuncture on anxiety and depression in unmarried patients with polycystic ovarian syndrome: secondary analysis of a pilot randomised controlled trial. *Acupunct Med* 2019;37:40-46.

[33] Zhou QZ, Peng XH, Wu QF, et al. [Effect of electroacupuncture on the expression of corticotropin releasing hormone (CRH) and CRHR 1 mRNA in paraventricular nucleus of hypothalamus in stress-induced anxiety rats]. *Zhen Ci Yan Jiu* 2008;33:372-376.

[34] Zhang J, Qin S, Zhou Y, Meng L, Su H, Zhao S. A randomized controlled trial of mindfulness-based Tai Chi Chuan for subthreshold depression adolescents. *Neuropsychiatr Dis Treat* 2018;14:2313-2321.

[35] Zhou M, Liao H, Sreepada LP, Ladner JR, Balschi JA, Lin AP. Tai Chi Improves Brain Metabolism and Muscle Energetics in Older Adults. *J Neuroimaging* 2018;28:359-364.

[36] Zhou JW, Zhang AR, Qiu L, et al. [Cognitive impairment in earthquake brain injury treated with comprehensive program of acupuncture and rehabilitation: a randomized controlled trial]. *Zhongguo Zhen Jiu* 2014;34:105-109.

[37] Sun R, Yang Y, Li Z, Li Y, Cheng S, Zeng F. Connectomics: a new direction in research to understand the mechanism of acupuncture. *Evid Based Complement Alternat Med* 2014;2014:568429.

[38] Cai H, Liang Q, Ge G. Gypenoside Attenuates beta Amyloid-Induced Inflammation in N9 Microglial Cells via SOCS1 Signaling. *Neural Plast* 2016;2016:6362707.

[39] Ye Q, Zhu YI, Ye S, et al. Gypenoside attenuates renal ischemia/reperfusion injury in mice by inhibition of ERK signaling. *Exp Ther Med* 2016;11:1499-1505.

[40] Chan HY, Stanton LW. A pharmacogenomic profile of human neural progenitors undergoing differentiation in the presence of the

traditional Chinese medicine NeuroAiD. *Pharmacogenomics J* 2016;16:461-471.

[41] Chen CL, Young SH, Gan HH, et al. Chinese medicine neuroaid efficacy on stroke recovery: a double-blind, placebo-controlled, randomized study. *Stroke* 2013;44:2093-2100.

[42] Heurteaux C, Gandin C, Borsotto M, et al. Neuroprotective and neuroproliferative activities of NeuroAid (MLC601, MLC901), a Chinese medicine, in vitro and in vivo. *Neuropharmacology* 2010;58:987-1001.

[43] Young SH, Zhao Y, Koh A, et al. Safety profile of MLC601 (Neuroaid) in acute ischemic stroke patients: A Singaporean substudy of the Chinese medicine neuroaid efficacy on stroke recovery study. *Cerebrovasc Dis* 2010;30:1-6.

[44] Wu X, Kaminga AC, Dai W, et al. The prevalence of moderate-to-high posttraumatic growth: A systematic review and meta-analysis. *J Affect Disord* 2019;243:408-415.

[45] Jang S, Jang BH, Ko Y, et al. Herbal Medicines for Treating Metabolic Syndrome: A Systematic Review of Randomized Controlled Trials. *Evid Based Complement Alternat Med* 2016;2016:5936402.

[46] Liu S, Wang XD, Wang Y, et al. Clinical and neuroimaging characteristics of Chinese dementia with Lewy bodies. *PLoS One* 2017;12:e0171802.

[47] Hu X, Teng S, He J, et al. Pharmacological basis for application of scutellarin in Alzheimer's disease: Antioxidation and antiapoptosis. *Mol Med Rep* 2018;18:4289-4296.

[48] Zhou Y, Li W, Han LF, et al. [Identification of Chinese Traditional Medicine Cistanches Herba from Different Places by HPLC-ESI-MS and FTIR Methods]. *Guang Pu Xue Yu Guang Pu Fen Xi* 2015; 35:1056-1061.

[49] Qiu Y, Chen M, Su M, et al. Metabolic profiling reveals therapeutic effects of Herba Cistanches in an animal model of hydrocortisone-induced 'kidney-deficiency syndrome'. *Chin Med* 2008;3:3.

[50] Xu C, Jia X, Xu R, Wang Y, Zhou Q, Sun S. Rapid discrimination of Herba Cistanches by multi-step infrared macro-fingerprinting combined with soft independent modeling of class analogy (SIMCA). *Spectrochim Acta A Mol Biomol Spectrosc* 2013;114:421-431.

[51] Zhou K. [The New Selected Chinese Medicine Associated Prescriptions]. *Hunan Science and Technology Press* 2010.

[52] Gu W, Shen XY, Zhou JJ, et al. [Distribution characteristics and correlation analysis of inorganic elements in Alismatis rhizoma and rhizospheric soils in different habitats]. *Zhong Yao Cai* 2012; 35:1893-1897.

[53] Zhou J, Xie J, Yan X. Encyclopedia of Tradiontal Chinese Medicines – Molecular Structures, Pharmacological Activities, Natural Resources and Applications. *Springer-Verlag Berlin Heidelberg* 2011.

[54] Zhou X, Ren Q, Wang B, Fang G, Ling Y, Li X. Alisol A 24-Acetate Isolated from the Alismatis Rhizoma Improves Hepatic Lipid Deposition in Hyperlipidemic Mice by ABCA1/ABCG1 Pathway. *J Nanosci Nanotechnol* 2019;19:5496-5502.

[55] Zheng Y, Li J, Wu J, et al. Tetrahydroxystilbene glucoside isolated from Polygonum multiflorum Thunb. demonstrates osteoblast differentiation promoting activity. *Exp Ther Med* 2017;14:2845-2852.

[56] Li JB, Zhao HY, Zhao YJ, et al. [Effects of Chinese herbal medicine Yiqi Huayu Bushen Recipe on expressions of aggrecan and type X collagen mRNAs in cells from degenerated human intervertebral discs]. *Zhong Xi Yi Jie He Xue Bao* 2011;9:1138-1144.

[57] Zhou YB, Yu JE, Wu J, et al. [Effects of Chinese herbal medicine Bushen Gubiao Recipe on toll-like receptor 4 and CD4(+)CD25(+)foxp3(+) regulatory T cells in mice with recurrent respiratory tract infections]. *Zhong Xi Yi Jie He Xue Bao* 2010; 8: 1053-1059.

[58] Zhu X, Zhou Y, Xu Q, Wu J. Traditional Chinese medicine Jianpi Bushen therapy suppresses the onset of pre-metastatic niche in a

murine model of spontaneous lung metastasis. *Biomed Pharmacother* 2017;86:434-440.

[59] Fang L, Zheng Q, Yang T, et al. Bushen Yisui Capsule ameliorates axonal injury in experimental autoimmune encephalomyelitis. *Neural Regen Res* 2013;8:3306-3315.

[60] Guo MD, Zhou WQ, Wei Y. [Clinical curative effect of Shenxiong Bushen Capsule and its effect on the quality of life of patients with Vascular dementia]. *Zhongguo Zhong Xi Yi Jie He Za Zhi* 2010;30:593-597.

[61] Zhu YC, Lin L, Zhou XL, Li RF, Hou LP. [Effect of Bushen Tongdu Capsule on RANK/RANKL/OPG pathway of collagen induced arthritis rats]. *Zhongguo Zhong Xi Yi Jie He Za Zhi* 2014;34:1487-1491.

[62] Chow DS, Horenstein CI, Canoll P, et al. Glioblastoma Induces Vascular Dysregulation in Nonenhancing Peritumoral Regions in Humans. *AJR Am J Roentgenol* 2016;206:1073-1081.

[63] Zips D, Adam M, Flentje M, et al. Impact of hypoxia and the metabolic microenvironment on radiotherapy of solid tumors. Introduction of a multi-institutional research project. *Strahlenther Onkol* 2004;180:609-615.

[64] Hadjiabadi DH, Pung L, Zhang J, et al. Brain tumors disrupt the resting-state connectome. *Neuroimage Clin* 2018;18:279-289.

[65] Harris RE, Ichesco E, Cummiford C, et al. Brain Connectivity Patterns Dissociate Action of Specific Acupressure Treatments in Fatigued Breast Cancer Survivors. *Front Neurol* 2017;8:298.

[66] Li X, He Y, Hou J, Yang G, Zhou S. A Time-Programmed Release of Dual Drugs from an Implantable Trilayer Structured Fiber Device for Synergistic Treatment of Breast Cancer. *Small* 2019:e1902262.

[67] Pattinson CL, Gill JM, Lippa SM, Brickell TA, French LM, Lange RT. Concurrent Mild Traumatic Brain Injury and Posttraumatic Stress Disorder Is Associated With Elevated Tau Concentrations in Peripheral Blood Plasma. *J Trauma Stress* 2019;32:546-554.

[68] Liu G, Yin T, Kim H, et al. Structure-activity relationship studies on Bax activator SMBA1 for the treatment of ER-positive and triple-negative breast cancer. *Eur J Med Chem* 2019;178:589-605.

[69] Vinayak S, Tolaney SM, Schwartzberg L, et al. Open-Label Clinical Trial of Niraparib Combined With Pembrolizumab for Treatment of Advanced or Metastatic Triple-Negative Breast Cancer. *JAMA Oncol* 2019.

[70] Samboju V, Philippi CL, Chan P, et al. Structural and functional brain imaging in acute HIV. *Neuroimage Clin* 2018;20:327-335.

[71] Ortega M, Brier MR, Ances BM. Effects of HIV and combination antiretroviral therapy on cortico-striatal functional connectivity. *AIDS* 2015;29:703-712.

[72] Hattab S, Guiguet M, Carcelain G, et al. Soluble biomarkers of immune activation and inflammation in HIV infection: impact of 2 years of effective first-line combination antiretroviral therapy. *HIV Med* 2015;16:553-562.

[73] Choi JY, Zhou J, Giles M, et al. Predictors and outcomes of HIV-infected antiretroviral-naive patients with discordant responses to combination antiretroviral treatment in Asian and Australian populations: results from APHOD. *J Acquir Immune Defic Syndr* 2011;57:e13-15.

[74] Shibata A, McMullen E, Pham A, et al. Polymeric nanoparticles containing combination antiretroviral drugs for HIV type 1 treatment. *AIDS Res Hum Retroviruses* 2013;29:746-754.

[75] Crowell TA, Fletcher JL, Sereti I, et al. Initiation of antiretroviral therapy before detection of colonic infiltration by HIV reduces viral reservoirs, inflammation and immune activation. *J Int AIDS Soc* 2016;19:21163.

[76] Zheng YH, Zhang CY, He Y, et al. The preliminary efficacy of interferon-alpha and ribavirin combination treatment of chronic hepatitis C in HIV-infected patients. *Chin Med J (Engl)* 2005;118:1195-1200.

[77] Zhou J, Sirisanthana T, Kiertiburanakul S, et al. Trends in CD4 counts in HIV-infected patients with HIV viral load monitoring

while on combination antiretroviral treatment: results from The TREAT Asia HIV Observational Database. *BMC Infect Dis* 2010;10:361.

[78] Barbieri A, Quagliariello V, Del Vecchio V, et al. Anticancer and Anti-Inflammatory Properties of Ganoderma lucidum Extract Effects on Melanoma and Triple-Negative Breast Cancer Treatment. *Nutrients* 2017;9.

[79] Jeong JJ, Kim B, Kim DH. Ginsenoside Rh1 eliminates the cytoprotective phenotype of human immunodeficiency virus type 1-transduced human macrophages by inhibiting the phosphorylation of pyruvate dehydrogenase lipoamide kinase isozyme 1. *Biol Pharm Bull* 2013;36:1088-1094.

[80] Rios-Fuller TJ, Ortiz-Soto G, Lacourt-Ventura M, et al. Ganoderma lucidum extract (GLE) impairs breast cancer stem cells by targeting the STAT3 pathway. *Oncotarget* 2018;9:35907-35921.

[81] Zhou J, Jaquet A, Bissagnene E, et al. Short-term risk of anaemia following initiation of combination antiretroviral treatment in HIV-infected patients in countries in sub-Saharan Africa, Asia-Pacific, and central and South America. *J Int AIDS Soc* 2012;15:5.

[82] Liang H, Ruan H, Ouyang Q, Lai L. Herb-target interaction network analysis helps to disclose molecular mechanism of traditional Chinese medicine. Sci Rep 2016;6:36767.

Chapter 7

SUMMARY OF MULTIPARAMETRIC IMAGING RESULTS

ABSTRACT

A summary of multiparametric imaging findings and correlations with clinical data in previous chapters 2-5 are listed in Tables in this chapter. Some proposed and reviewed traditional Chinese medicines for neurodegenerative disease treatment in chapter 6 were summarized in Table as well. A neurobiology model of the pathological processes such as accumulation of tau and amyloid (Aβ), demyelination and dysfunction in specific regions with the neurodegenerative diseases was proposed.

SUMMARY

A summary of significant imaging findings including 12 imaging features at function, structure and molecular scales of four neurodegenerative diseases in previous chapters 2-5 are listed in Tables 1. Significant correlations between homotopic imaging with clinical data in PTSD patients are listed in Table 2, and significant correlations between homotopic imaging with neurocognitive data in MS patients are listed in Table 3 respectively in this chapter. Some proposed and reviewed traditional Chinese medicine (TCM) for neurodegenerative disease treatment in chapter 6 are summarized in Table 4.

Our results included specific regions and neuronal networks, various neuropathological burdens, multiple structural and microstructural connectivities and function-related changes; different and some opposite small-worldness properties of four neurodegenerative diseases. A simple illustration of multiparametric imaging is shown in Figure 1. For example, one of the mostly involved regions (dysfunction found in eight imaging metrics including four neuronal network fcMRI disconnectivities, hypoactivity, higher VMHC, higher tau and amyloid), vmPFC plays an important role in PTSD related syndrome; and was associated with most of the clinical data (8 out of 12 tests as listed in Table 2). Likewise, the hippocampus was presented in most memory-associated tests based on VMHC results; and was found dysfunctional in MCI patients compared to controls based on six imaging features (three fcMRI disconnectivities, hypoactivity, lower FA and higher tau).

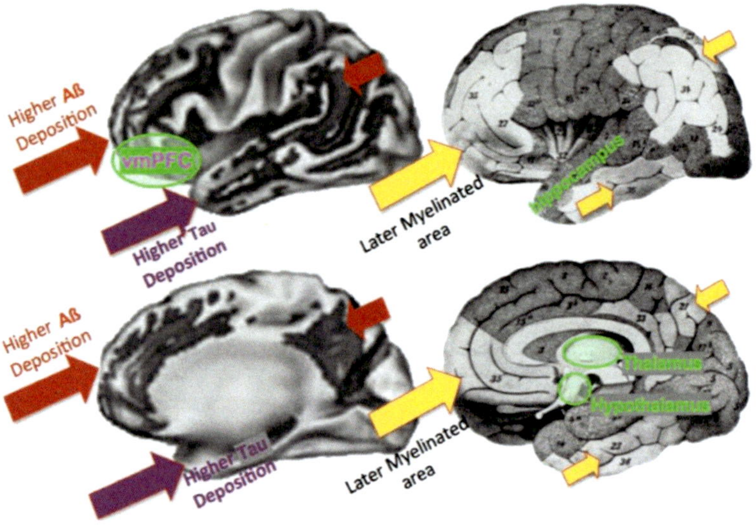

Figure 1. The neuropathological processes such as accumulation of tau, amyloid (Aβ) and demyelination are the common underlying causes of neurodegeneration involved in brain injuries after accident, stress, dementia or inflammation. The regions with higher amyloid and tau burdens co-localized with the later myelinated areas (arrows) that are more vulnerable to injuries such as the medial prefrontal and posterior cingulate cortices, hippocampus, and hypothalamus. The specific regions and networks of interest reported including vmPFC, hypothalamus, thalamus, hippocampus (green) in the PTSD/MTBI/MCI/MS patients had been visualized with multiparametric images at function, structure and molecular scales in this book.

Table 1. Significant brain regional alterations (P < 0.01) in neurodegenerative diseases from our results presented in chapters 2-5

Metrics	PTSD	MTBI	MCI	MS
fcMRI default mode network (Figures 7, 12, 17, 22 in Chapter 2)	Lower in MPFC, PCC, temporal cortex Higher in vmPFC, thalamus, and SMA	Lower in the PCC and parietal regions; Higher in MPFC	Lower in hippocampus, MPFC and PCC; Higher in inferior temporal, OFC and small visual regions	Lower in MPFC, middle cingulate and SMA; Higher in small inferior temporal and occipital cortices
fcMRI hypothalamus Figures 8, 13, 18, 23 for PTSD, MTBI, MCI and MS patients respectively in Chapter 2	Lower in small temporal regions, midbrain (pons, substantia nigra), right Broca's area, MA, SMA; Higher in vmPFC, hippocampus & visual cortex	Lower in temporal, MPFC, PCC, right inferior parietal, SMA; Higher in visual cortex and MA	Lower in large temporal regions including amygdala & hippocampus, vmPFC, SMA, cerebellum; Higher in DLPFC, cingulum, parietal regions	Lower in midbrain, inferior temporal, SMA, cerebellum; Higher in midbrain, small regions in striatum and MA
fcMRI hippocampus (Figures 9, 14, 19, 24 in Chapter 2)	Lower in vmPFC and temporal cortex; Higher in bilateral parietal and cerebellar regions	No significant differences	Higher in temporal cortex including hippocampus, hypothalamus, MPFC; Lower in DLPFC, parietal, cingulum and cerebellum	Lower in occipital, superior parietal and SMA; Higher in MPFC, PCC, hippocampus and inferior parietal
fcMRI thalamus (Figures 10, 15, 20, 25 in Chapter 2)	Lower in subcortical temporal, premotor and somatosensory cortices; Higher in vmPFC, cerebellum and inferior OFC	Lower in frontal and temporal cortices; higher in visual and parietal cortices (thalamic segment 4,7)	Higher in inferior temporal cortex, PCC and midbrain; Lower in DLPFC and parietal regions	Lower in MPFC, insula, ventral striatum, small temporal and visual regions, higher in superior parietal and precuneus
fALFF (Figures 11, 16, 21, 26 in Chapter 2)	Lower in vmPFC, amygdala, hippocampus, and superior temporal regions; Higher in inferior parietal, angular and occipital regions	Lower in the thalamus, scattered regions in MPFC, occipital, and temporal cortex	Lower in MPFC, temporal cortex including hippocampus and superior segment, parietal; Higher in inferior temporal cortex MA and SMA	Lower in somatosensory, superior parietal, visual cortex and temporal-occipital junction; higher in vmPFC, temporal, MFC, and frontal, striatum

Table 1. (Continued)

Metrics	PTSD	MTBI	MCI	MS
VMHC (Figures 1, 4, 5, 6 in Chapter 3)	Lower in the thalamus, temporal, parietal occipital, and frontal white matter areas, thalamic radiation and optic radiation, striatum; Higher in vmPFC	Lower in DLPFC, hippocampus, small regions in temporal and visual; Higher in vmPFC and small middle cingulate	Lower in cuneus and MPFC; Higher in distributed regions in the temporal, visual, motor and parietal cortices	Lower in primary frontal, temporal, and visual cortices; higher in anterior insular, thalamus, striatum, cerebellum, and inferior temporal regions
SMW (Table 4 in Chapter 4)	Lower local efficiency & small-worldness (SMW); Higher global efficiency	Lower global efficiency; Higher local efficiency	Lower local efficiency and small-worldness; Higher global efficiency	No significant differences
DTI-FA (Figure 1, 3, 4, 5 in Chapter 4)	Lower in forceps major and corticospinal; Higher in thalamic radiation and left uncinate fasciculus	Lower in frontal, occipital and corpus callosum (diffuse axonal injuries)	Lower in tracts that connect the hippocampus such as bilateral fornix and left cingulum	Lower in corpus callosum, cingulate bundles, optic radiation and short U-fibers (lowest in lesions)
Morphometry (Table 1 in Chapter 4)	Lower cortical thickness, surface area and volume in the pars opercularis, anterior cingulate, postcentral, and temporal pole as well as transverse temporal regions	No significant differences at initial visit; global atrophy, anterior cingulate and isthmus WM, precuneal GM atrophy at 1-year follow-up	Lower cortical thickness in the posterior cingulate and inferior temporal in stables; middle frontal, posterior cingulate, fusiform in converters	Lower brain parenchymal fraction; regional GM atrophy in PCC, inferior parietal, MPFC, thalamus, basal forebrain, primary somatosensory cortex
Tau (mainly for PTSD and MCI (Chapter 5)	Higher in vmPFC, cingulate, precuneus, lingual, parietal perculum, hippocampus, thalamus, putamen, intracalcarine cortex and planum polare in PTSD		Higher in hippocampus , temporal fusiform, frontal operculum cortex, cuneus, and accumbens in MCI patients. (Figures 1-4 for tau, and Figures 5,6 for amyloid in Chapter 5)	
Amyloid (PTSD& MCI)	Higher in vmPFC, scattered regions in temporal, occipital and inferior parietal cortices in PTSD		Higher global cerebral cortex, regional MPFC and PCC in MCI compared to controls (Figure 5, 6 in Ch. 5)	
FDG	Global hypometabolism in PTSD		Global hypometabolism in MCI	

vmPFC = ventromedial prefrontal cortex; PCC = posterior cingulate; MPFC = medial prefrontal cortex; SMA = supplementary motor area, MA = motor area; OFC = orbitofrontal cortex; DLPFC = dorsolateral prefrontal cortex; WM = white matter; GM = gray matter.

Chapter 2 for four fcMRI and fALFF results; Chapter 3 for VMHC; Chapter 4 for DTI, Morphometry and SMW; Chapter 5 for Molecular Imaging including tau amyloid and FDG tracers.

Table 2. Summary of significant correlations between VMHC imaging and clinical data for PTSD data cohort in Chapter 3

Clinical Tests	Correlations Between Homotopic Images and Clinical Tests of PTSD Patients ($P < 0.01$) with results shown in Figures 7-10 in Chapter 3
CAPS	Negative in temporal, subcortical putamen, uncinate fasciculus, thalamic radiation, optic radiation and parietal regions; Positive only in small regions in vmPFC and cerebellum
NPI	Positive in hippocampus, anterior temporal, occipital, cuneus and parietal/motor regions; Negative in small scattering regions in the cerebellum and occipital cortex.
CES	Positive in insula, anterior and middle cingulate, dorsolateral, medial prefrontal cortices and cerebellum; Negative in small areas in inferior temporal, inferior parietal and occipital cortices
GDS	Positive in gyrus rectus; Negative in superior portion of vmPFC, medial prefrontal and dorsolateral prefrontal cortices, cerebellum, thalamus, superior temporal and occipital regions
ADAS	Negative in large areas of orbitofrontal cortex including vmPFC, temporal cortex including hippocampus, midbrain, thalamic radiation and motor area; Positive in small occipital region
TICS	Negative in vmPFC, medial prefrontal cortex, temporal region including fusiform, and small region in supplementary motor cortex; Positive in the temporo-parietal junction, thalamus, small regions in posterior cingulate, cuneus and motor area
MMSE	Positive in the vmPFC, temporal, occipital, angular and dorsolateral prefrontal cortex
AFQT Total	Positive in the medial prefrontal and orbito-prefrontal including vmFPC, temporal cortex including hippocampus, small region in posterior cingulated, subcortical caudate and thalamus; Negative in the cerebellum, temporo-occipital conjunction, and cuneus.
AFQT Object	Positive in the posterior temporal cortex including fusiform, occipital cortex, cuneus, posterior cingulate, medial prefrontal region; Negative in the inferior temporal region, hypothalamus, motor and dorsolateral prefrontal regions
AFQT Mathematics	Positive in small regions in the vmPFC, angular, fusiform and cuneus; Negative in medial prefrontal and dorsolateral prefrontal cortices, small inferior temporal and caudate regions
AFQT Spatial Orientation	Positive in the vmPFC, motor area and inferior temporal regions as well as thalamus; Negative in the small region of posterior temporal, parietal, medial frontal, insular and cuneus cortices
AFQT Vocabulary	Positive in small regions of temporal and parietal cortices, precuneus and post-central area

CAPS = clinician-administered PTSD scale; NPI = neuropsychological inventory; CES = Combat Exposure Scale; GDS = Geriatric Depression Scale; ADAS = Alzheimer's Disease Assessment Scale of cognitive function; TICS = Telephone interview for Cognitive Status; MMSE = Mini-Mental State Examination; AFQT = Armed Forces Qualification Tests with four categories.

In conclusion, the various neuroimaging results indicated that regions with higher amyloid and tau burdens co-localized with the later myelinated areas (detected with abnormal VMHC) that are more vulnerable to injuries such as the medial prefrontal and posterior cingulate cortices, hippocampus, and hypothalamus. Functional connectivity networks from these specific regions including DMN, vmPFC, hypothalamus, thalamus, hippocampus measured with fcMRI also identified abnormal functional connectivity and activity deficits in the four neurodegenerative diseases with high sensitivities.

Table 3. Summary of significant correlations between VMHC imaging and neurocognitive tests for MS data cohort in Chapter 3

Neurocognitive Tests	Correlations Between Homotopic Images and neurocognitive Tests of MS Patients (P<0.01) with results shown in Figures 11-14 in Chapter 3
DKEFS Color, Word, Switching and Instant Switching; Verbal Fluency, Fatigue; Depression	Dorsolateral prefrontal, cerebellum and posterior cingulate for Fatigue score with positive correlation; but negative correlation with the Depression score. Primary and associate visual cortices including V3 and V4 for color, Broca's and Wernicke's regions for word processing and verbal fluency; vmPFC and superior temporal, visual, motor areas for mental flexibility and visual attention; dorsolateral prefrontal cortex for executive function.
Digital Span; SDMT; Trial B Test; CE Error, Time; PASAT	Orbitofrontal, medial and dorsolateral prefrontal cortices, and cuneus for information processing accuracy and time, working memory and executive function; visual cortex, cerebellum, temporal and medial prefrontal cortices for visual-perception, auditory and sustained attention.
RCFT Copy, Delayed Recall (DR), Immediate Recall (IR); CVLT Learning and Memory, DR, IR	Significant correlations in the anterior and superior temporal segments for the delayed recall that might encode memory information functionality, Broca's and orbitofrontal areas for immediate recall; temporal cortex including hippocampus, posterior cingulate, dorsolateral and medial prefrontal regions as well as Wernicke's area for executive function, verbal learning and memory encoding and recall.
Expanded Disability Status Scale (EDSS)	Negative correlations included cuneus, unimodal auditory cortex (e.g., Wernicke's area), vmPFC, medial prefrontal, inferior temporal and motor areas; positive correlations were mainly in the medial temporal, dorsolateral frontal, premotor and primary visual cortices.

DKEFS=Delis-Kaplan Executive Function Scale; SDMT= Symbol Digit Modalities Test; CE= cognitive examination; PASAT=Paced Auditory Serial Addition Test; RCFT=Rey-Osterrieth Complex Figure Test; CVLT= California Verbal Learning Test

The abnormal microstructural and morphological findings had further validated the local regional and pathway injuries in brain in these diseases. The additional tight associations between imaging findings and most clinical tests suggested these multiparametric data could be used as noninvasive, *in vivo*, valid and composite biomarkers for distinguishing the neurodegenerative diseases from each other and from controls with high specificities.

Table 4. Summary of reviewed Traditional Chinese Medicine (TCM) for neurodegenerative disease treatment in Chapter 6

Diseases	**PTSD**	**MTBI**	**MCI**	**MS**
Traditional Chinese Medicine	Gastrodin Morinda officinalis , Albiflorin, Electroacupuncture and Tai Chi Chuan	Tai Chi Chuan, Gypenoside and NeuroAid	Scutellarin, Cistanches herba, Rhizoma Alismatis, Polygonum multiflorum thumb and Bushen capsules (BSCs)	*Ginkgo biloba,* Gastrodin

About the Author

Yongxia Zhou

Scientist, Department of Radiology and Biomedical Engineering, University of Southern California and Columbia University

Yongxia Zhou is a medical imaging scientist, specialized in MRI neuroimaging and neurosciences applications. She had completed my PhD from University of Southern California in Biomedical imaging in 2004 and had been trained and worked as neuroimaging scientists in several prestigious institutes including Columbia University, New York University and University of Pennsylvania and NIH. Her research focuses on multi-modal neuroimaging including using MRI/PET and EEG instrumentation as well as the integration of these multi-modal to make the best usage of each modality and to help interpreting underlying co-existing patho-physiological for better disease diagnosis and treatment. Her specific interests in MRI technology include brain mapping of blood flow, oxygen saturation and extraction fraction and metabolism as well as vascular reactivity assessment with fMRI activity/connectivity and arterial spin labeling (ASL)-based blood flow measures. She had published 6 books and 5 book chapters, about 100 papers and abstracts in well-known international journals and conferences. She has been serving as several journal and international conference reviewers including JMRI, JCBFM, HBM, AJNR, PlosOne, ISMRM and ICAD.

INDEX

A

aberrant connections, 131
abnormal connectivity, 8, 19, 59, 103
absolute clustering coefficient, 111
absolute shortest-path length, 111
abuse, vii, 4, 7, 16, 17, 26, 108, 122
accumbens, 74, 75, 93, 112, 136, 138, 170
acupuncture, 152, 154, 160
acute HIV infection (AHI), 156
adrenal cortex, 5
age, 26, 27, 28, 47, 55, 67, 70, 71, 75, 76, 94, 102, 108, 119, 123, 145
age-related, 119
aging, 11, 13, 57, 63, 92, 93, 103, 115, 126, 127, 140, 141, 142, 143, 147, 149, 154
aging effects, 92, 93
aging-related diseases, 11, 154
Albiflorin, 153, 173
alpha waves, 8
Alzheimer's disease (AD), vii, x, xiv, 2, 11, 27, 28, 46, 54, 62, 93, 95, 102, 108, 118, 126, 130, 132, 152, 155
Alzheimer's disease assessment scale (ADAS), xiii, 27, 66, 68, 69, 82, 84, 94, 101, 131, 171
Alzheimer's Disease Assessment Scale–Cognitive (ADAS-Cog), 27, 68, 101
Alzheimer's Disease neuroimaging initiative (ADNI), 27, 28, 29, 57, 110, 132, 138, 142, 143
amygdala, ix, xii, 6, 14, 24, 37, 39, 45, 52, 53, 56, 62, 109, 136, 139, 141, 147, 153, 169
amyloid, vi, vii, x, xiv, xv, xvi, 4, 10, 11, 20, 47, 54, 60, 63, 100, 122, 126, 128, 129, 130, 131, 132, 137, 138, 140, 141, 142, 144, 145, 147, 148, 149, 154, 160, 162, 167, 168, 170, 172
amyloid accumulation, xv, 130, 133, 137, 138, 141
amyloid aggregation, 131
amyloid deposition, x, xv, 63, 130, 132, 137, 138, 140, 141, 142
amyloid load, 47
amyloid neurotoxicity, 131
amyloid pathology, vii, 11, 100, 144
amyloid plaque(s), viii, 11, 54, 132, 137, 142
anger symptoms, 108
angular, 37, 53, 82, 85, 86, 119, 139, 141, 169, 171
animal models, 154

anterior cingulate, xiv, 6, 108, 111, 113, 119, 170
anterior cingulated cortex, 6
anti-inflammatory, 152
antioxidant, 154
anti-oxidative, 152, 153
anti-phase synchronization, 51
anti-radical effects, 153
antiretroviral treatment (ART), 15, 58, 156, 164, 165
anxiety, 6, 16, 26, 39, 50, 61, 70, 71, 97, 98, 102, 109, 119, 122, 148, 153, 160
appetite, 9
appetite regulation, 9
Armed Forces Qualification Test (AFQT), xiii, 27, 66, 68, 69, 82, 85, 86, 87, 94, 171
arousal, vii, 5, 9, 10, 14, 59, 67
arterial stiffness, 141
atlas, 133, 136
atrophies, 8, 111, 120
attention control, 140
attentional control, 5
attentional processing, 156
auditory, 21, 27, 53, 68, 72, 73, 76, 77, 81, 88, 90, 140, 172
autoimmune diseases, 92
autoimmune inflammation process, 152
autoimmune inflammatory disease, 12
avoidance, vii, 4, 5, 67
axonal cytoskeleton damage, 131
axonal injury, 8, 51, 121, 153, 163

B

basal forebrain, 39, 51, 113, 120, 170
baseline, 116, 138
blood oxygen level-dependent (BOLD), 24, 155
blood-brain barrier damage, 141
Boston naming test, 27, 68
Braak, x, xv, 130, 133, 135, 136, 140, 142, 144
Braak stage(s), x, xv, 130, 133, 135, 136, 140, 142
Braak staging, xv, 130, 136, 140
brain abnormalities, viii, 8
brain atrophy, viii, 12, 120
brain changes, x, xiv, 6, 10, 107, 109, 152
brain disorders, 152, 154
brain injury, 8, 26, 51, 60, 61, 145, 160
brain integrity, 156
brain networks, 6, 24, 55, 59, 155
brain parenchymal fraction, 113, 170
brain region-specific, viii, xi, 1, 3
brain tumors, 155, 163
brain waves, 8
breast cancer survivors, 155
Brodmann areas (BA), 13, 77, 80, 97, 101, 110
BSCs therapy, 155
Bushen capsules (BSCs), 155, 173

C

California Verbal Learning Test (CVLT), 70, 71, 101, 172
callosal degeneration, 95
cancer, x, 152, 155, 156, 157, 163, 164, 165
cardiovascular function, 154
cART, 156
category switching, 70
caudate, 19, 36, 39, 73, 75, 82, 83, 85, 86, 109, 123, 136, 171
Centipeda minima, 154
central executive network (CEN), 6, 25, 33, 34
central nervous system, 9, 111, 157
central nervous system (CNS), 9, 15, 111, 157
cerebellum, xiii, 9, 32, 34, 35, 36, 40, 45, 46, 47, 48, 49, 51, 53, 54, 55, 66, 80, 81,

82, 83, 84, 85, 87, 88, 93, 113, 118, 132, 134, 137, 169, 170, 171, 172
cerebral blood flow, 18, 153
cerebral cortex, vii, 11, 47, 58, 103, 155
cerebrovascular injury, 141
challenging diseases, x, xv, 151, 152, 155
chemotherapy, 156
chinese herbal medicine (CHM), 152, 154, 159, 162
chinese herbs, 152
chinese medicine, 152, 159, 161
chronic, viii, 8, 12, 16, 18, 62, 67, 98, 105, 116, 127, 130, 140, 141, 144, 152, 154, 156, 158, 164
chronic distress, 154
chronic stress, 67, 130, 141
chronic TBI, 8
chronic traumatic encephalography (CTE), 140
cingulate, xiii, xv, 36, 40, 45, 47, 53, 55, 58, 61, 66, 71, 74, 75, 78, 82, 83, 93, 112, 116, 117, 119, 120, 121, 130, 134, 136, 139, 141, 169, 170, 171
cingulate bundles, 116, 117, 119, 170
cingulum, x, xiv, 7, 54, 55, 91, 92, 107, 108, 109, 113, 114, 115, 118, 119, 121, 124, 169, 170
Cistanches herba, 154, 173
clinical assessment, 69
clinical data, x, xi, xii, xvi, 1, 2, 4, 65, 67, 96, 167, 168, 171
Clinical Dementia Rating (CDR), 27, 100
clinical symptom, viii, ix, xi, xiii, 1, 2, 3, 10, 12, 24, 25, 39, 56, 66, 69, 94, 96, 155
clinical symptom relevance, 2
clinical symptoms, ix, xi, xiii, 10, 12, 24, 25, 39, 56, 66, 94, 96, 155
clinician-administered PTSD scale (CAPS), xiii, 27, 66, 69, 81, 83, 94, 171
closed head injury, vii, 26
clustering coefficient, 118
cognition, 124, 149, 157
cognitive ability, 153
cognitive dysfunction, 8, 104, 130, 131
cognitive examination (CE), 70, 172
cognitive function, xiii, 52, 64, 66, 94, 104, 106, 154, 155, 171
cognitive reserve, 67
Combat Exposure Scale (CES), 27, 68, 69, 82, 83, 171
Combination ART (cART), 156
comorbid, vii, 14, 52, 67, 97, 98, 100, 109, 126, 131, 143, 147
complementary and alternative medicine (CAM), 152, 153, 157
complex pathophysiologies, 152
composite biomarkers, 173
composite memory score, 138
comprehensive imaging features, viii, 142
comprehensive template, 30
connectome, 90, 91, 92, 105, 120, 127, 148, 163
conscious perception, 8
contralateral hemisphere, 155
corpus callosum (CC), x, xiv, 6, 12, 72, 90, 91, 95, 108, 109, 113, 116, 117, 118, 119, 121, 122, 170
correlation matrix, 110
cortical thickness, xiv, 4, 108, 110, 111, 112, 118, 119, 120, 121, 170
cortical thinning, vii, 11, 112, 120, 126
corticospinal, x, xiv, 94, 107, 108, 113, 114, 118, 119, 121, 154, 170
corticospinal system, 154
corticospinal tract, 94, 108, 113, 114, 118
cortico-striatal network, 156
corticotropin releasing hormone (CRH), 5, 160
cortisol hypersecretions, 7
cuneus, xiii, 45, 66, 74, 76, 77, 78, 79, 82, 83, 84, 85, 86, 87, 88, 90, 93, 95, 136, 137, 138, 141, 170, 171, 172

D

default mode network (DMN), viii, ix, xi, 1, 3, 6, 7, 8, 10, 11, 15, 23, 24, 25, 29, 30, 31, 32, 35, 38, 44, 46, 47, 48, 50, 53, 54, 55, 56, 61, 93, 141, 155, 156, 169, 172
delayed recall, 70, 89, 172
Delis-Kaplan executive function scale (D-KEFS), 70
dementia, xi, 2, 3, 11, 20, 24, 52, 55, 56, 60, 67, 97, 105, 120, 126, 145, 147, 154, 157, 161, 163, 168
demyelinating, viii, 12, 21, 152
demyelinating disease, viii, 12, 21, 152
demyelination, x, xvi, 10, 92, 119, 121, 131, 144, 153, 167, 168
density of myelin, 91, 92
depression, xiii, 6, 25, 26, 39, 50, 53, 58, 60, 66, 70, 87, 88, 94, 95, 100, 102, 104, 105, 109, 143, 153, 157, 160, 171, 172
detection specificity, 2
diagnosis, vii, viii, x, xi, 1, 2, 3, 17, 28, 95, 96, 127, 142, 175
diagnosis accuracy, viii, 2, 142
diffuse axonal injury, x, xiv, 8, 10, 17, 18, 51, 108, 116, 119, 120, 121, 125
diffuse axonal injury (DAI), x, xiv, 8, 10, 17, 18, 51, 108, 116, 119, 120, 121, 125
diffusion tensor imaging (DTI), viii, ix, xiv, 4, 11, 12, 72, 90, 91, 99, 104, 107, 108, 109, 110, 113, 119, 122, 123, 124, 126, 170
diffusivities, 113
digit span, 69, 71
disease mechanism, x, 1, 2, 3, 141, 152, 153
disease progression, viii, 12, 153
distance-based conductivity, 93
dorsal attention network (DAN), 24, 32, 33, 156
dorsolateral prefrontal, ix, xiii, 6, 44, 45, 46, 49, 55, 66, 67, 73, 78, 82, 83, 84, 85, 86, 87, 88, 89, 93, 95, 108, 170, 171, 172
dorsolateral prefrontal cortex, 6, 44, 49, 55, 67, 82, 85, 87, 88, 108, 170, 171, 172

E

EDSS score, xiii, 66, 89, 90, 95
effective treatments, 152
electroacupuncture (EA), 14, 101, 154, 160, 173
emotion regulation, 6, 53, 109, 154
endothelial function, 153
energy imbalance, 153
enhanced brain function, 156
enhanced single prolonged stress (ESPS), 153
entorhinal, viii, xv, 11, 130, 136, 139, 140, 141
environmental monitoring, 25
episodic and working memory, 155
episodic memory, 5, 6, 54, 63
Everyday Cognition (ECog), 27
excitotoxicity, 153
executive function(s), xiii, xiv, 4, 5, 16, 38, 55, 66, 67, 70, 87, 88, 89, 95, 102, 108, 121, 123, 140, 156, 172
Expanded Disability Status Scale (EDSS), xiii, 28, 66, 70, 89, 90, 95, 172
exposure, vii, 16, 67, 102, 124, 156, 171
extracellular amyloid, 141

F

fatigue, vii, xi, xiii, 10, 24, 25, 26, 28, 39, 43, 50, 53, 56, 66, 70, 87, 88, 95, 102, 104, 153, 172
fatigue severity scale, 10, 70, 102

fcMRI, ix, xi, xv, 3, 6, 8, 12, 23, 24, 25, 29, 30, 31, 32, 34, 35, 36, 37, 38, 41, 43, 44, 45, 46, 47, 48, 49, 50, 51, 52, 53, 54, 55,
FDG-glucose, viii, x, xv, 129, 132
fear extinction, 109
fears, 6
Fluoro-2-deoxyglucose (FDG), vi, viii, x, xv, 4, 15, 20, 52, 60, 62, 63, 129, 130, 132, 139, 141, 147, 162, 170
fMRI, viii, xi, 3, 7, 8, 11, 12, 15, 23, 24, 29, 44, 51, 61, 62, 67, 96, 99, 109, 110, 118, 120, 155, 175
follow-up, 70, 71, 111, 120, 139, 141, 170
formation of glial scars, 153
fornix, x, xiv, 107, 113, 115, 119, 121, 127, 170
fractional amplitude of low frequency fluctuation (fALFF), xi, 3, 11, 23, 24, 25, 32, 34, 35, 37, 38, 42, 43, 44, 46, 47, 49, 50, 52, 53, 54, 55, 169, 170
fractional anisotropy (FA), x, xiv, 4, 12, 63, 72, 90, 91, 95, 107, 108, 109, 110, 113, 114, 115, 116, 117, 118, 119, 121, 122, 132, 145, 168, 170
frame displacement (FD), 31
freesurfer, 110, 111
front eye field (FEF), 32
frontal, vii, ix, x, xi, xiii, xiv, 8, 23, 34, 35, 38, 41, 42, 43, 50, 52, 53, 54, 55, 56, 66, 67, 73, 74, 76, 77, 79, 80, 81, 86, 90, 93, 94, 95, 99, 108, 112, 115, 116, 117, 118, 119, 121, 131, 136, 137, 138, 156, 169, 170, 171, 172
frontal operculum cortex, 138, 170
frontal pole, 116, 117
FSL, 31, 41, 42, 43, 71, 72, 110, 113, 115, 133
functional activity, ix, xi, 11, 12, 23, 37, 46, 49, 54, 55, 56
functional adaptation, viii, 11
Functional Assessment Questionnaire (FAQ), 27
functional connectivity, ix, xi, 3, 6, 10, 11, 12, 16, 17, 18, 20, 21, 23, 24, 38, 43, 50, 51, 54, 58, 59, 64, 90, 95, 99, 100, 103, 104, 105, 110, 151, 155, 156, 157, 164, 172
functional connectivity based MRI (fcMRI), ix, xi, xv, 3, 6, 8, 12, 23, 24, 25, 29, 30, 31, 32, 34, 35, 36, 37, 38, 41, 43, 44, 45, 46, 47, 48, 49, 50, 51, 52, 53, 54, 55, 56, 71, 151, 168, 169, 170, 172
functional coordination, xii, 24, 56, 93, 94
functional homotopy, xii, 65, 68, 95, 99
functional hyperactivity, 94
functional integration, xii, 65, 67
functional network, ix, xi, xiv, 8, 23, 25, 39, 51, 56, 107, 109
functional rerouting, 54
functional voxel-mirrored homotopic correlation (VMHC), ix, xii, xiii, 3, 12, 65, 66, 67, 68, 71, 72, 73, 75, 76, 77, 80, 81, 82, 87, 88, 89, 90, 92, 93, 94, 95, 96, 168, 170, 171, 172
fusiform, 72, 73, 75, 77, 82, 83, 84, 85, 86, 112, 136, 138, 170, 171

G

gain energy, 152
gamma waves, 8
Ganoderm lucidum, 156
Gastrodin, 153, 159, 173
Geriatric Depression Scale (GDS), xiii, 27, 66, 68, 69, 82, 84, 94, 100, 171
Ginkgo, 153, 159, 173
Ginkgo biloba tablets (GBT), 153
Glasgow Coma Scale (GCS), vii, 26
glial activation, 156
glioblastoma, 155, 163
global cerebral cortex, 138, 170
global efficiency, x, xiv, 10, 108, 110, 117, 118, 120, 121, 170

global hypometabolism, 139, 141, 170
glucose metabolism, 132
graph-theory, x, xiv, 3, 31, 107, 110
greater survival rate, 156
Gypenoside, 154, 160, 173

H

herb, 153, 154, 160, 165
heteromodal, 72, 73, 76, 77, 81, 91, 92
heteromodal association, 72
highly active antiretroviral therapy (HAART), 156
high-specificity, 140
hippocampal, viii, ix, x, xi, xiv, xv, 7, 11, 14, 16, 23, 31, 33, 36, 43, 45, 46, 48, 49, 52, 53, 55, 56, 63, 104, 105, 107, 108, 119, 121, 130, 131, 140, 148, 154, 155, 158
hippocampal atrophy, 7, 63, 131
hippocampal cingulum, x, xiv, 108, 119, 121
hippocampal fcMRI, ix, xii, 24, 33, 36, 43, 45, 46, 48, 49, 52, 53, 55, 56
hippocampal formation, 31
hippocampal neurogenesis, 154
hippocampal volume, 7, 16
hippocampus, ix, xi, xii, xiii, xv, 1, 3, 6, 7, 11, 12, 13, 14, 15, 16, 19, 24, 25, 30, 32, 33, 35, 37, 44, 45, 46, 53, 54, 56, 59, 66, 67, 73, 75, 78, 82, 83, 84, 85, 89, 93, 98, 103, 113, 115, 130, 131, 132, 134, 135, 136, 138, 140, 141, 145, 148, 153, 154, 168, 169, 170, 171, 172
histogram, 91, 92
homotopic connections, ix, xii, 66, 73, 74, 76, 78, 79, 81, 82, 83, 93
homotopic connectivity, 81, 82, 87
homotopy imaging, ix, xii, 65, 68
Human Connectome Project, 72, 100
human immunodeficiency virus (HIV), 15, 58, 155, 156, 164, 165
hyperarousal, vii, 4, 5, 6
hyperarousal symptoms, 5, 6
hyperconnectivity, 16, 38, 98
hypervigilance, 5, 7, 119
hypoconnectivity, 6, 38, 53
hypocretin, 9, 14, 19
hypometabolism, x, xv, 8, 18, 52, 130, 141, 142
hypometabolism of glucose, x, xv, 130, 141
hypothalamic, vii, viii, ix, xi, xv, 5, 8, 9, 10, 13, 14, 19, 23, 31, 33, 35, 36, 39, 40, 43, 45, 47, 48, 51, 53, 54, 55, 56, 61, 67, 98, 130, 131, 140
hypothalamic connectivity, xi, 10, 19, 24, 39, 51, 56, 61
hypothalamic dysfunction, vii, 10, 51
hypothalamic fcMRI, 10, 33, 35, 36, 39, 40, 45, 47, 48, 53, 54, 55
hypothalamic injury, viii, 8, 10
hypothalamic reactivity, 51
hypothalamic RSN, 33, 51
hypothalamic-pituitary-adrenal (HPA), 5, 6, 10, 13, 67, 98, 100, 131, 143
hypothalamus, ix, xi, xii, 1, 3, 5, 7, 9, 10, 12, 14, 24, 25, 30, 31, 39, 40, 43, 46, 51, 53, 55, 56, 58, 82, 85, 131, 133, 135, 160, 168, 169, 171, 172

I

imaging biomarkers, viii, x, xi, 12, 23, 56, 142
immediate recall, 89, 172
immune system activation, 131
impaired episodic autobiographical recall, 6
in post concussion syndrome, 10
in vivo, 10, 62, 100, 152, 161, 173
independent component analysis (ICA), 30, 31, 38

inducible NO syntheses (iNOS), 153
inferior fronto-occipital fasciculus, 113, 114, 118
inferior longitudinal fasciculus, 113, 114, 118
inferior orbitofrontal, 49, 53, 55, 82, 84
inferior parietal cortex, 39, 45, 139, 141
inferior parietal lobe (IPL), xv, 11, 32, 76, 79, 130, 137, 141
inferior temporal, 7, 34, 44, 46, 47, 54, 55, 81, 82, 83, 85, 86, 87, 90, 94, 112, 133, 134, 135, 136, 140, 169, 170, 171, 172
inferior temporal cortex, 34, 46, 54, 112, 136, 140, 169
inferior temporal gyrus, 112
inflammation, xii, 24, 57, 67, 146, 148, 153, 156, 160, 164, 168
information processing, xii, xiii, 65, 66, 67, 69, 88, 95, 109, 140, 172
insomnia, 7, 95, 105
insula, xiii, 6, 49, 66, 82, 83, 93, 136, 156, 169, 171
interference switching, 70
interhemispheric, xii, 12, 65, 67, 71, 81, 90, 93, 94, 95, 96, 99, 104, 105
interhemispheric connections, 94
interhemispheric connectivity, 67
interhemispheric coordination, 94, 99
internal capsule, 109, 114
intracalcarine cortex, 72, 134, 135, 170
intracellular tau, 11, 141
intrusions, vii, 4
intrusive trauma recollection, 6
ion accumulation, 153
irritability, 5, 7
isthmus white matter, 71, 111, 120

L

lack of motivation, vii, 10
large-scale samples, x, 1, 2
later myelinated areas, 168, 172
lesion probability map (LPM), 116, 117
lesions, 9, 29, 116, 119, 170
limbic system, 52
lingual, 134, 135, 136, 137, 170
local efficiency, x, xiv, 108, 111, 117, 118, 120, 121, 170
local neuronal injuries, 53
local regional activity, xi, 23, 25
longevity, 152
longitudinal, 11, 13, 14, 17, 21, 61, 64, 71, 103, 119, 120, 138, 139, 143
longitudinal changes, 11
longitudinal date, 139
loss of consciousness, 26, 109, 123

M

Magnetization-prepared rapid acquisition gradient-echo (MPRAGE), 29, 31, 110
magnetoencephalography (MEG), 7
major forceps, x, xiv, 107, 108, 113, 114, 118, 121
MATLAB, 133
MCI converters, 112, 118
MCI subtypes, 120
mean diffusivity, 109, 128
mechanical stress, 131
medial prefrontal cortex (MPFC), xii, 11, 24, 25, 29, 32, 37, 38, 40, 44, 45, 46, 49, 50, 53, 54, 56, 76, 79, 84, 88, 131, 139, 140, 169, 170, 171
medial temporal lobe (MTL), 11
memory, xii, xiv, 2, 6, 7, 16, 20, 24, 25, 52, 53, 54, 55, 56, 63, 70, 89, 93, 94, 98, 103, 108, 109, 119, 121, 123, 125, 130, 140, 141, 146, 147, 153, 154, 157, 158, 159, 168, 172
memory and learning, 154
memory encoding, 25, 172
memory scores, 94

mental flexibility, 38, 70, 87, 88, 172
metabolic dysfunction, 153
metabolic stress, 131
metabolism, xiv, 4, 5, 9, 13, 14, 59, 62, 124, 129, 132, 143, 160, 175
metabolism dysfunction, xiv, 129, 132
microstructural, v, ix, xiv, 4, 7, 10, 51, 95, 96, 105, 107, 109, 110, 111, 119, 121, 122, 123, 142, 148, 168, 173
microstructural changes, 95
microstructure, viii
microstructure integrity, viii
midbrain, 35, 46, 47, 53, 54, 55, 82, 84, 115, 169, 171
mild cognitive impairment (MCI), viii, ix, x, xii, xiii, xiv, xv, 11, 19, 20, 24, 25, 27, 28, 29, 44, 45, 46, 47, 53, 54, 56, 59, 60, 65, 66, 68, 72, 73, 76, 79, 93, 94, 96, 101, 103, 107, 108, 109, 112, 113, 115, 118, 119, 120, 121, 126, 129, 130, 132, 138, 139, 140, 141, 142, 147, 148, 149, 154, 162, 168, 169, 170, 173
mild traumatic brain injury (MTBI), vii, ix, x, xi, xii, xiii, xiv, 1, 8, 10, 14, 17, 19, 23, 25, 26, 28, 31, 38, 39, 40, 41, 42, 43, 50, 51, 52, 56, 59, 60, 61, 62, 64, 65, 66, 67, 68, 69, 70, 71, 72, 73, 75, 77, 78, 93, 94, 96, 101, 103, 104, 107, 108, 109, 111, 116, 118, 119, 120, 121, 122, 123, 125, 129, 146, 157, 168, 169, 170, 173
mind reading, 152
Mini-Mental State Examination (MMSE), xiii, 27, 66, 68, 69, 82, 85, 94, 112, 171
molecular, vi, viii, x, xi, xiv, xv, 1, 2, 3, 7, 20, 62, 108, 129, 130, 132, 133, 138, 140, 141, 142, 144, 145, 146, 147, 162, 165, 167, 168, 170
molecular imaging, x, xv, 2, 3, 129, 130, 132, 138, 140, 141
Montreal Cognitive Assessment (MOCA), 27
Montreal Neurological Institute (MNI), 29, 31, 77, 80, 133
mood, 5
morphological, x, xiv, 7, 107, 109, 110, 115, 121, 142, 173
morphological quantifications, 110
morphology, viii
morphometry, v, 4, 107, 110, 111, 119, 170
motivation, 5, 55
motor area, 48, 55, 81, 82, 84, 86, 87, 88, 90, 134, 137, 170, 171, 172
motor function, 89, 154
MPFC, 11, 25, 29, 32, 38, 50, 53, 54, 131, 139, 169, 170
multiparametric, vi, viii, x, xvi, 1, 2, 3, 7, 11, 61, 132, 152, 167, 168, 173
multiparametric imaging, x, xvi, 1, 2, 7, 11, 132, 152, 167, 168
multiparametric neuroimaging, viii, 3
multiple lesions, viii, 12
multiple sclerosis (MS), viii, ix, x, xii, xiii, xiv, 2, 12, 18, 20, 21, 24, 25, 28, 47, 48, 49, 50, 55, 56, 60, 64, 65, 66, 68, 69, 70, 72, 73, 80, 81, 87, 88, 89, 90, 91, 92, 93, 94, 95, 96, 99, 102, 103, 104, 105, 106, 107, 108, 109, 113, 116, 117, 118, 119, 120, 121, 125, 127, 131, 132, 146, 152, 153, 158, 159, 161, 167, 168, 169, 170, 172, 173
myelin, ix, xii, 3, 12, 65, 68, 72, 76, 90, 91, 92, 93, 95, 99, 100, 103, 108, 120, 126, 131, 152, 159
myelin contents, 120
myelin depth, 91, 92
myelin distribution, 76, 93
myelin map, ix, xii, 65, 68, 72, 91, 92, 95, 100
myelin mapping, 72
myelin maturation age, 108
myelin repair, 131
myelin sheath, 92

N

negative alterations in cognition and mood, vii, 4
negative connectivity, 32, 33, 34, 51
nerve-regulating factors, 154
neural plasticity, 153
neural underpins, 2, 96
NeuroAid, 154, 161, 173
neurobiology, viii, x, xi, xvi, 1, 3, 4, 167
neurobiology model, x, xvi, 167
neurocognitive, v, ix, xi, xii, 1, 2, 4, 13, 50, 65, 66, 68, 69, 71, 81, 87, 88, 90, 96, 97, 146, 167, 172
neurocognitive dysfunction, 50
neurocognitive function, xi, 1, 2, 13, 51
neurodegeneration, xi, 1, 2, 20, 95, 127, 131, 132, 146, 148, 152, 168
neurodegenerative disease, viii, ix, x, xi, xii, xiv, xv, xvi, 1, 2, 3, 4, 11, 12, 24, 25, 56, 65, 68, 95, 96, 107, 109, 120, 121, 129, 130, 132, 140, 141, 142, 151, 152, 153, 155, 167, 168, 169, 172, 173
neuroendocrine system, 5
neurofibrillation tangle (NFT), 131, 141
neuroimaging, v, vi, viii, x, xi, xv, 1, 2, 3, 4, 8, 12, 13, 20, 21, 22, 27, 52, 57, 59, 60, 61, 62, 68, 96, 98, 100, 106, 121, 122, 125, 126, 127, 130, 142, 143, 144, 146, 147, 148, 149, 151, 152, 159, 160, 161, 162, 172, 175
neuroimaging quantifications, x, xv, xvi, 130, 142, 151, 152
neuroimaging techniques, viii, 4, 8, 12
neuroinflammation, xiv, 95, 129, 132, 148, 153
neuronal activation, 3, 7, 12, 32, 37, 53
neuronal activity, 8, 10, 34, 62, 141
neuronal damage, 153
neuronal network, ix, xi, xii, 3, 23, 24, 25, 52, 55, 56, 168
neurons, 5, 8, 9, 19, 155
neuropathological burden(s), viii, xv, 4, 10, 130, 140, 168
neuropathological examination, 131
neuropathological hallmarks, 130
neuropathological processes, 168
neuropeptide dysregulation, vii, 10
neuroplasticity, 50, 54, 104, 152
neuroplasticity enhancement, 152
neuroprotective, 152, 153, 154, 161
neuropsychological inventories, xi, 1, 2
neuropsychological inventory (NPI), 68, 69, 81, 83, 171
neuropsychological symptoms, 95
neuropsychological tests, ix, xii, 26, 27, 65, 68, 69, 95
neuroregeneration, 95
neurorestorative, 154
nitric oxide (NO), 153
NO bioavailability, 153
noninvasive, 152, 173
non-specific binding, 133
normal appearing brain tissue abnormalities, viii, 12
nutrition, 152, 153

O

object discrimination, 68, 94
occipital, ix, x, xii, xiii, xiv, xv, 6, 7, 24, 34, 35, 37, 41, 42, 43, 47, 48, 49, 51, 53, 55, 56, 66, 72, 73, 74, 75, 76, 77, 78, 79, 81, 82, 83, 84, 85, 90, 93, 94, 108, 113, 114, 116, 118, 119, 121, 130, 131, 134, 136, 137, 138, 141, 156, 169, 170, 171
occipital cortex, 6, 35, 43, 49, 51, 53, 82, 83, 85, 90, 136, 156, 171
optic radiation, ix, x, xiii, xiv, 66, 73, 74, 81, 83, 93, 94, 108, 116, 117, 119, 121, 170, 171
or loss of consciousness, vii, 26

or stress disorder, xi, 24, 56
orbitofrontal, xv, 32, 33, 34, 44, 53, 54, 55, 82, 84, 88, 89, 130, 133, 135, 140, 170, 171, 172
orbitofrontal cortex, 32, 33, 44, 82, 84, 170, 171
orexin, 5, 9, 14, 19, 51
orexin neurons, 5, 9
oxidative and metabolic stress, 153

P

Paced Auditory Serial Addition Test (PASAT), 70, 71, 172
pain, 6, 13, 98, 100
pallidum, xiii, 66, 80, 93, 137, 138
paracentral motor areas, 46, 54
parahippocampal cortex, 156
parietal, ix, xii, xiii, xv, 7, 11, 34, 36, 37, 38, 40, 43, 44, 45, 46, 48, 49, 53, 54, 55, 66, 73, 74, 75, 76, 77, 79, 81, 82, 83, 86, 87, 91, 93, 94, 113, 120, 130, 131, 134, 135, 136, 137, 138, 139, 140, 141, 169, 170, 171
parietal cortex, 46, 136
parietal perculum, 134, 170
pars opercularis, xiv, 108, 111, 119, 170
pathogenesis of neurodegeneration, 154
pathomechanisms, xi, 7, 23, 56
pathophysiological mechanisms, 8
pathway damage, 53
PCC, 6, 11, 25, 29, 32, 38, 50, 53, 54, 131, 139, 169, 170
Pearson correlation, 38, 67, 110
peri-hypothalamic regions, 33, 40, 51
peripheral benzodiazepine receptor, 132
periventricular regions, 116, 117
PET, viii, 4, 18, 20, 27, 52, 60, 62, 63, 131, 132, 144, 146, 147, 148, 149, 162, 175
phosphorylated-tau, 154
pituitary, 5
planum polare, xv, 74, 130, 134, 135, 140, 170
polygonum multiflorum thumb, 155, 173
positive connectivity, 32, 33, 34, 40
post concussion symptom scale (PCSS), 70, 71, 102
post concussion syndrome (PCS), xi, 24, 26, 52, 56, 118
post traumatic stress disorder (PTSD), vii, ix, x, xi, xii, xiii, xiv, xv, 2, 4, 5, 6, 7, 10, 13, 14, 15, 16, 17, 23, 25, 27, 28, 29, 35, 36, 37, 52, 56, 59, 60, 62, 65, 66, 67, 68, 69, 72, 73, 74, 75, 76, 81, 82, 83, 93, 94, 96, 97, 98, 99, 101, 107, 108, 109, 111, 112, 113, 114, 115, 117, 118, 119, 120, 121, 122, 124, 129, 130, 131, 132, 133, 134, 135, 136, 137, 138, 139, 140, 141, 142, 145, 152, 153, 167, 168, 169, 170, 171, 173
posterior cingulate (PCC), xii, xiii, xv, 6, 11, 19, 24, 25, 29, 30, 32, 33, 34, 35, 38, 43, 44, 46, 50, 53, 54, 56, 59, 66, 73, 82, 84, 85, 87, 88, 89, 95, 103, 112, 113, 120, 130, 131, 135, 137, 138, 139, 140, 141, 168, 169, 170, 171, 172
posterior cingulate cortex (PCC), 6, 11, 25, 29, 32, 38, 50, 53, 54, 120, 131, 139, 169, 170
posttraumatic, vii, 8, 13, 14, 15, 16, 17, 26, 59, 60, 62, 66, 96, 97, 98, 100, 101, 122, 123, 124, 125, 127, 143, 144, 145, 146, 148, 161, 163
Post-traumatic stress disorder (PTSD), vii, ix, x, xi, xii, xiii, xiv, xv, 1, 2, 4, 5, 6, 7, 10, 13, 14, 15, 16, 17, 23, 25, 27, 28, 29, 35, 36, 37, 52, 56, 59, 60, 62, 65, 66, 67, 68, 69, 72, 73, 74, 75, 76, 81, 82, 83, 93, 94, 96, 97, 98, 99, 100, 101, 104, 106, 107, 108, 109, 111, 112, 113, 114, 115, 117, 118, 119, 120, 121, 122, 123, 124, 126, 129, 130, 131, 132, 133, 134, 135, 136, 137, 138, 139, 140, 141, 142, 144,

145, 147, 148, 149, 152, 153, 160, 167, 168, 169, 170, 171, 173
posttraumatic symptoms, 8, 26
post-traumatic symptoms, 7
post-traumatic symptoms, 50
preclinical stages, viii, 11
precuneal gray matter, 111, 120
precuneus, xv, 49, 55, 86, 87, 130, 134, 135, 136, 137, 140, 169, 170, 171
prefrontal, xii, xiii, xv, 5, 6, 7, 24, 30, 33, 35, 36, 39, 43, 46, 47, 49, 50, 51, 52, 53, 54, 55, 66, 67, 72, 73, 77, 81, 82, 83, 84, 85, 86, 87, 88, 89, 90, 91, 92, 93, 95, 109, 113, 119, 120, 130, 137, 138, 141, 153, 157, 168, 170, 171, 172
prefrontal cortex, 6, 49, 52, 53, 55, 67, 109, 153, 170
primary age-related tauopahty, 11
primary cortices, xiii, 66, 81
primary motor areas, 44
primary somatosensory cortex, 113, 120, 170
primary visual cortex, 76, 93
problems with appetite and arousal, vii, 10
problems with sleep, vii, 10
processing speed and accuracy, 4
psychiatric disorder, vii, xii, 4, 26, 65, 67, 104, 111
PTSD+TBI, 131
public health, vii, 8

Q

quality of life, 19, 95, 97, 104, 156, 163

R

rapid eye movement (REM), 9
ratio of standard uptake value (SUVR), 132, 133, 137, 139
reaction time, 109
reactive oxygen species (ROS), 153, 155
red Ginseng, 156
re-experiencing, vii, 4, 67, 93
regional distributions, 92
regional parcellation, 133
regional quantification, xv, 76, 130, 132, 140
regions of interest (ROI(s)), 3, 29, 31, 39, 75, 110, 112, 113, 114, 115, 118, 132, 133, 134, 135, 136, 137, 138, 139
region-specific, 140
relapsing-remitting (RR), 28, 124, 128, 153
relative betweenness centrality, 118
relative clustering coefficient, 111
relative path length, 111
relaxed awareness, 8
relay central station, vii
resting state networks, 15, 24, 58, 156
resting-state fMRI (RS-fMRI), xi, 3, 11, 12, 23, 24, 27, 28, 29, 31, 32, 41, 42, 43, 46, 51, 54, 71, 104, 105, 156
Rey-Osterrieth Complex Figure Test (RCFT), 70, 71, 90, 91, 172
Rhizoma Alismatis, 154, 173
ROS accumulation, 155
rostral anterior cingulate (rAC), 71
RS-fMRI, xi, 3, 11, 12, 23, 24, 27, 28, 29, 31, 32, 41, 42, 43, 46, 51, 54, 71

S

sagittal stratum, 113, 115
salience network, 6, 108, 156
Scutellarin (SC), 6, 17, 61, 106, 121, 125, 126, 147, 154, 157, 159, 173
secondary progressive MS (SPMS), 153
self-relevance, 25
senile dementia, 155
sensitivity, viii, xv, 3, 55, 95, 130, 142
sensitivity and specificity, viii, xv, 130, 142
sensorimotor, 12, 21, 25, 127, 155

shearing forces, 131
short U-fibers, 116, 117, 119, 170
significant correlations, xi, xiii, 24, 56, 66, 88, 89, 94, 95, 109, 138, 139, 141, 167, 171, 172
sleep disturbance, xi, 10, 24, 56
sleep regulation, 9
sleep/wake cycles, 5, 10
small-worldness (SMW), x, xiv, 4, 31, 107, 108, 110, 117, 118, 120, 121, 168, 170
somatosensory, xiii, 36, 49, 53, 55, 66, 72, 73, 76, 77, 81, 91, 92, 93, 134, 137, 169
somatosensory cortex, 49, 53, 55, 76, 91, 92, 93
spatial correspondence, 93
spatial orientation, 68, 87, 94
specificity, 155
spinal cord injury, 153, 159
stables, 112, 118, 120, 170
stress, v, vi, xii, 4, 5, 7, 13, 14, 15, 16, 17, 23, 24, 57, 59, 60, 61, 62, 65, 66, 67, 94, 96, 97, 98, 100, 101, 104, 107, 119, 122, 123, 124, 125, 126, 127, 129, 131, 140, 143, 144, 145, 146, 148, 154, 160, 164, 168
stress disorder, xii, 13, 14, 15, 16, 17, 24, 57, 60, 62, 66, 96, 97, 98, 100, 101, 122, 123, 124, 125, 127, 140, 143, 144, 145, 146, 148
stress-related changes, 119
striatum, xiii, 13, 48, 50, 55, 66, 73, 74, 81, 93, 94, 145, 169, 170
structural connectivity, xii, xiv, 12, 65, 72, 90, 95, 107, 109, 156
structural connectivity abnormalities, xiv, 107, 109
structural reorganization, viii, 11
structure, x, xiv, 1, 108, 164, 167, 168
subcortical, xiii, xv, 7, 36, 66, 73, 74, 76, 77, 78, 81, 82, 83, 85, 93, 94, 124, 130, 133, 137, 140, 142, 169, 171
subcortical area, xiii, 66, 73, 76, 77, 78, 93, 133, 137
subcortical thalamus, 133
substantia nigra, 35, 169
superior longitudinal fasciculus, 108, 113, 114, 115, 118
superior parietal lobe, 33, 49, 138
supplementary motor area(s), 35, 44, 45, 47, 48, 53, 54, 55, 170
surface area, xiv, 4, 108, 110, 111, 112, 119, 121, 170
sustained attention, xiii, 66, 70, 88, 95, 172
Symbol Digit Modalities Test (SDMT), 69, 101, 172
symptomatology, 26, 123
systematic analyses, xii, 65, 68

T

Tai Chi, 152, 154, 158, 160, 173
Tai Chi Chuan, 152, 154, 160, 173
task-negative network, 31
tau, vi, viii, x, xiv, xv, xvi, 4, 10, 11, 20, 54, 63, 129, 130, 131, 132, 133, 134, 135, 136, 137, 138, 140, 141, 142, 144, 147, 148, 149, 158, 164, 167, 168, 170, 172
tau deposition, xv, 130, 133, 134, 135, 136, 137, 138, 140, 141
tau nucleation, 131
tau spreading, 141
tau tangle, viii, 11, 54, 131, 132, 142
tau tangles, viii, 11, 54, 131, 142
tau-crosslinked microtubules, 131
tauopathy, 60, 62, 100, 125, 131, 146, 147
TBSS, 110, 113, 115, 116, 117, 118, 132
TCM, xv, 151, 152, 153, 154, 156, 167, 173
Telephone interview for Cognitive Status (TICS), xiii, 66, 68, 69, 84, 94, 171
tempo-occipital conjunction, xiii, 66
temporal, vii, ix, x, xi, xii, xiii, xiv, xv, 7, 11, 18, 23, 32, 33, 35, 36, 37, 41, 42, 43,

45, 46, 49, 52, 53, 54, 55, 56, 66, 73, 74, 75, 76, 77, 78, 79, 80, 81, 82, 83, 84, 85, 86, 87, 88, 89, 90, 91, 92, 93, 94, 95, 108, 111, 112, 113, 114, 118, 119, 121, 130, 131, 134, 136, 137, 138, 139, 140, 141, 142, 149, 155, 169, 170, 171, 172
temporal cortex, 11, 32, 33, 36, 46, 53, 54, 82, 84, 85, 89, 112, 120, 121, 136, 138, 141, 169, 171, 172
temporal pole, xiv, 11, 108, 111, 119, 136, 170
temporal-occipital junction, 49, 55, 169
temporo-occipital, 82, 85, 89, 95, 112, 171
temporo-parietal junction, 6, 92
thalamic connectivity, xii, 24, 48, 55, 56
thalamic radiation, ix, xii, xiii, 66, 73, 74, 81, 82, 83, 84, 93, 94, 108, 113, 114, 118, 170, 171
thalamo-cortical, 8, 9, 10, 17, 41, 43, 52, 60, 118, 120
thalamo-cortical connections, 8, 10
thalamo-cortical connectivity, 10, 41, 52, 118
thalamo-cortical functional connectivity, 52
thalamo-frontal, 52
thalamo-temporal, 52
thalamo-thalamo fcMRI, 43, 52
thalamus, vii, ix, xi, xiii, 1, 3, 7, 8, 10, 13, 18, 19, 25, 30, 31, 33, 34, 35, 39, 41, 42, 43, 52, 53, 58, 62, 66, 73, 74, 75, 80, 81, 82, 84, 85, 86, 87, 93, 94, 113, 120, 132, 133, 134, 135, 136, 168, 169, 170, 171, 172
thalamus projections, 94
the temporo-parietal junction, 84, 171
the trail making test, 27, 68
therapeutic effects, x, xv, 151, 152, 161
therapeutic efficacy, viii, 153
therapeutic evidence, 151
therapeutic guidance, 6
therapy, 154, 157, 159, 163, 164
tissue injury, viii, 12
tract-based spatial statistics (TBSS), 21, 110, 113, 115, 116, 117, 118, 132
traditional Chinese medicine (TCM), x, xv, xvi, 144, 151, 152, 153, 154, 156, 157, 158, 161, 163, 165, 167, 173
traffic accident, vii, 4, 67, 96, 97, 99
Trail-Making Test A, 69
Trail-Making Test B (TMB), 69
translocator protein (TSPO), 132
transverse temporal, xiv, 108, 111, 112, 119, 170
traumatic accident, xii, 24, 51, 57
traumatic brain injury (TBI), vii, x, xv, 2, 8, 10, 13, 14, 17, 18, 19, 27, 50, 52, 60, 61, 62, 67, 96, 98, 99, 100, 103, 109, 122, 123, 124, 125, 126, 127, 128, 130, 131, 132, 133, 135, 137, 140, 141, 142, 144, 145, 146, 152, 154, 158
traumatic event, vii, 66, 67, 108
traumatic experience, 108
traumatic exposure, vii, 4
treatment effects, 152
treatment efficacy, xv, 151
treatment evaluations, x
tuberomamillary nucleus, 39

U

ultrastructure, 155
uncinate, x, xiv, 81, 83, 107, 109, 113, 114, 118, 121, 124, 170, 171
uncinate fasciculus, 81, 83, 109, 113, 114, 118, 124, 170, 171
unimodal association, 72

V

validation, xii, 2, 13, 59, 65, 68, 72, 90, 95, 96, 102, 106, 120, 121, 149
vascular inflammation, 152
ventral striatum (VST), 49, 169

ventral tegmental area (VTA), 9
ventromedial prefrontal cortex (vmPFC), ix, x, xii, xiii, xv, 6, 7, 15, 24, 35, 36, 37, 45, 48, 50, 53, 55, 56, 66, 67, 73, 74, 78, 81, 82, 83, 84, 85, 86, 87, 88, 90, 93, 94, 109, 130, 133, 134, 135, 137, 138, 140, 142, 168, 169, 170, 171, 172
verbal fluency, xiii, 66, 87, 88, 95, 172
veteran, 67, 109
visual attention, 69, 87, 88, 172
visual cortex, 32, 33, 75, 81, 88, 91, 92, 100, 169, 172
visual disturbances, 28
visual perception and attention, 4
visual-perception, xiii, 66, 88, 95, 172
VMHC, ix, xii, xiii, 3, 12, 65, 66, 67, 68, 71, 72, 73, 75, 76, 77, 80, 81, 82, 87, 88, 89, 90, 92, 93, 94, 95, 96, 168, 170, 171, 172
vmPFC, ix, x, xii, xiii, xv, 6, 7, 24, 35, 36, 37, 45, 48, 50, 53, 55, 56, 66, 67, 73, 74, 78, 81, 82, 83, 84, 85, 86, 87, 88, 90, 93, 94, 109, 130, 133, 134, 135, 137, 138, 140, 142, 168, 169, 170, 171, 172
volume, xiv, 4, 7, 17, 63, 64, 71, 103, 108, 110, 111, 112, 119, 121, 124, 139, 170
volumetry, x, xiv, 107, 109, 111, 112, 132, 139
voxel-based morphometry (VBM), 113
voxel-mirrored homotopic correlation (VMHC), ix, xii, xiii, 3, 12, 65, 66, 67, 68, 71, 72, 73, 75, 76, 77, 80, 81, 82, 87, 88, 89, 90, 92, 93, 94, 95, 96, 168, 170, 171, 172

W

warfare, vii, 4, 67
white matter (WM), xiii, xiv, 4, 8, 10, 20, 41, 43, 46, 60, 63, 66, 71, 73, 74, 93, 94, 103, 104, 107, 108, 109, 115, 116, 117, 119, 121, 122, 123, 124, 126, 127, 128, 131, 132, 141, 147, 149, 152, 162, 170
white matter atrophy, 10
white matter deterioration, 141, 152
white matter integrity, xiv, 4, 107, 108, 109, 119, 122, 123, 124, 127
white matter lesion load (WMLL), 20, 46, 60, 147, 162
white matter lesions, 132
working memory, xiii, 4, 5, 7, 54, 61, 66, 69, 71, 88, 95, 104, 172